Dash Diet Weight Loss Solution 2019

The Weight Loss Solution for Beginners with Meal Prep and Exquisite Recipes

***By:* Jason Heller**

Table of Contents

Introduction 1

DASH Diet 3

Chapter 2: Helpful Tricks and Tips 12

Chapter 3: Meal Program 24

Chapter 4: Breakfast Recipes 41

    Bacon Egg & Spinach Casserole 41

    Biscuits & Gravy 45

    Breakfast Tostadas 48

    Creamy Oatmeal 51

    Egg Salad 53

    Eggs Benedict 56

    Fruit Smoothie 59

    Green Smoothie 61

    Homemade Bacon 63

    Oatmeal Pancakes 67

    Sausage Patties 70

    Stuffed Potatoes 72

    Quiche Cups 75

Chapter 5: Lunch Recipes 78

    American Chopsuey 78

    Asian Chicken Wraps 81

    Baked Chicken 85

    Cheesy Mushroom Risotto 89

    Chicken Gyros 93

Chicken Salad 96
Fettuccine Alfredo 100
Fish Fillets 104
Fish Stew 106
Fried Rice 109
Mexican Salad 113
Minestrone Soup 116
Mushroom Fajitas 120
Orange Chicken 122
Veggie Jambalaya 126
Oven Baked Sea Bass 130
Quinoa Salad 132
Sloppy Joe Sandwich 136
Spaghetti with Vegetables 139
Tuna Salad 142
Turkey Panini 144
Turkey Tacos 146
Vegetable Soup 150
Zucchini Frittata 153

Chapter 6: Dinner Recipes 155

Baked Salmon 155
Beef Stroganoff 157
Black Bean Burgers 162
Chicken Kabobs 165
Crunchy Fried Chicken 169
Herbed Oven Roasted Veggies 171
Lintel Stew 174

Mashed Potatoes 176
Pumpkin Soup 179
Red Beans & Rice..182
Sesame Chicken 185
Thai Vegetable Curry.......................................188
Turkey Meatloaf...193
Veggie Lasagna 198
Vegetarian Chili 202
Vegetarian Pizza 206
Zesty Mushroom Soup 208

Chapter 7: Dressings, Sauces& Condiments 213

Avocado Dressing 213
Barbeque Sauce 215
Chicken Broth 217
French Dressing..220
Italian Dressing 222
Ketchup...224
Marinara Sauce 227
Mayonnaise...230
Mustard...232
Peanut Butter..234
Ranch Dressing 236
Soy Sauce 238
Taco Seasoning 241
Tartar Sauce 243
Thai Marinade 245
Thousand Island Dressing 247

Tzatziki Sauce 249
Vegetable Broth...251
Worcestershire Sauce 255
Yogurt Dressing 258

Chapter 8: Snacks and Desserts 260

Apple Crumb Cake Muffins 260
Carrot Dip..264
Cauliflower Rice...266
Fiesta Dip 269
Macaroni & Cheese 273
Mozzarella Sticks 276
Peanut Butter Bars...278
Potato Salad 282
Red Pepper Hummus......................................285
Rice Pudding 288
South American Guacamole 290
Stuffed Mushrooms 292
Tomato Salsa 296
Trail Mix 298

Conclusion..300

Index for the Recipes 301

Introduction

Congratulations on downloading your copy of the Dash Diet Weight Loss Solution: *The Weight Loss Solution for Beginners with Meal Prep and Exquisite Recipes.* I am excited that you have selected to take the venture into incorporating the DASH Diet plan into your life.

This book is specifically for beginners, but this does not mean that tried and true followers of the DASH Diet will not gain benefit from the information contained within. In fact, there are some sensational recipes that also have helpful tips included that may help to diversify your recipe box.

Knowing that time is an important resource for everyone, the recipes in this book are easy to make and do not take that much time. There is a guide for beginners of how to get started today as well as a detailed week-long meal plan that will be a fantastic guide to making the transition to the DASH Diet less stressful for you.

In following the meal plan and the recipes laid out for you as well as the tips to be successful, you will find that making this life-changing decision will be the best that you have made for you and your health. There is a variety of possibilities to use the information and recipes in this cookbook to make living on the DASH diet enjoyable.

There a few recipes with a few more steps to follow, but each recipe will provide you with an estimated preparation and cooking time, amount of servings, and a list of nutritional values including sodium, protein, fat, sugar, and calorie content. You will have everything that you will need using this cookbook to get started in bettering your health today.

There are plenty of books on the DASH Diet in the market today. Thanks again for choosing this one! Every effort was made to ensure that it is full of as much useful information as possible.

DASH Diet

Overview

Generally speaking, most people who are looking to start the DASH diet are people who suffer from high blood pressure themselves or have a family member that does.

Men are going to be more likely to have hypertension issues especially after the age of 45, and a significant amount of patients with diabetes will experience these symptoms as well. Also, put at risk are individuals who are overweight. However, hypertension can happen to anyone.

DASH is an acronym for Dietary Approaches to Stop Hypertension. The diet is centered on eating a balanced combination of lean meats, vegetables, whole grains and fruits, and keeping sodium intake between two-thirds and one tablespoon of salt per day depending on the reasons for starting the diet and the results you are seeking.

The DASH diet also focuses on keeping fats, added sugars and red meat to a lower level. As with all diets, there is a happy medium for keeping true to the diet. Do not get stressed out as it will be shown in this book how to get started and give you guidelines to follow that will be easy to incorporate into your daily life.

When you experience the symptoms of hypertension for extended amounts of time, you are more at risk for heart disease, kidney issues, and higher glucose levels leading to diabetes. You also are at a higher risk of early mortality as this chart shows.

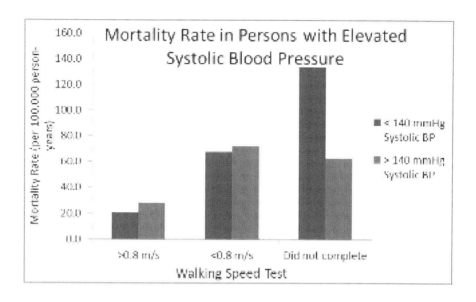

However, following the simple to understand guidelines of the DASH Diet will help to bring your blood pressure numbers to a more manageable level and help you to be healthier in the long run, bringing your chances of living a much more fulfilling life for you.

When you work towards your goals on the DASH Diet, you will start to see the results rather quickly which will help you to keep your willpower working towards your personal goals.

Do you know where you personally need to be in better health? Chances are you know what your current blood pressure and glucose levels are at. Knowing this information, you will know how hard you will need to work to achieve your personal goals.

This easy to read chart shows what levels you want to achieve for your blood pressure and glucose levels to be at optimum health.

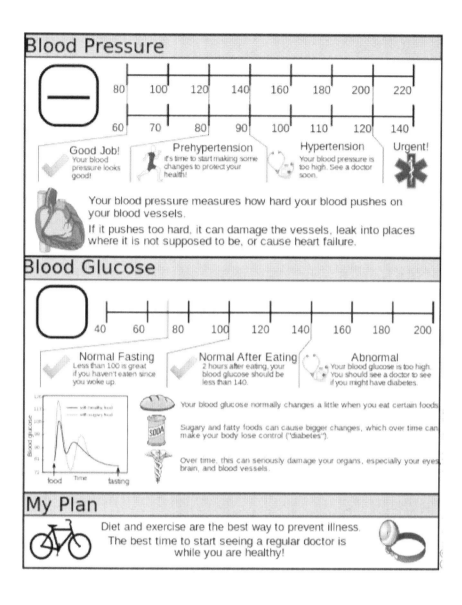

Advantages of the DASH Diet

Other than the obvious benefit of the DASH diet for

lowering your blood pressure, you may experience weight loss, a reduced risk for certain cancers, diabetes, and kidney and heart-related issues to name a few. Considering these are major headlines when it comes to American health, it is worth taking a look as to how the DASH Diet can benefit you personally.

As for the blood pressure impacts, it has been found that the salt intake has the largest result in lowering your numbers to a healthy level. Even the individuals who follow the DASH diet but do not partake in a strict lowering of sodium intake saw benefits from the diet.

However, when the salt was kept at the recommended levels of a teaspoon of salt a day or less, there was a higher impact on the blood pressure calculations dropping. So, if you are on the DASH diet because you or someone you love suffers from high blood pressure, restricting the salt intake would see the most beneficial results.

The impact of the DASH Diet on blood pressure levels has been extensively studied. The result which has been continuously found is that individuals following the restricted sodium consumption saw a drop in their blood pressure numbers within two weeks. So, it is worth trying something different to be able to feel the benefits in such a short period of time.

But do not fret if you do not see rapid results. It did not take overnight to get to this point in your life, and it will take an effort to reverse what has been done. However, the reward will be well worth the effort that you put into making these positive changes in your life.

Even though weight loss is not the main goal of the DASH diet, it comes as an extra bonus because you are making healthier food choices by cutting out processed, high fat, and sugary foods, which, in turn, will likely help you shed pounds.

It is important to note that not all participants will

lose weight as it depends on your daily activities and the macronutrients that you consume. However, because the sodium intake is being decreased, you will see the blood pressure being lowered regardless.

As mentioned before, there is a decreased risk of cancers to include breast and colon cancers. This is due to the number of vegetables and fruits you would be eating rather than empty calorie sweets and processed foods.

Because you are putting whole foods into your body, you will feel a natural boost in your energy levels and your mental clarity will begin to sharpen. You will also feel less hungry as you are not filling your body with empty calories that most Americans crave with the sugary and processed snacks.

For sufferers of Type 2 diabetes, the DASH Diet will assist you with your insulin resistance, making sure there are no spikes and dips in your glucose levels.

Because sugars are kept lower naturally in the diet, this limits the number of sugar crashes you will experience during the day.

Because the DASH Diet specifically impacts the blood pressure, this will have a positive benefit to people who suffer from heart-related issues. As a result, your blood pressure will be reduced, and it will put less stress on your heart bringing better overall health.

You may also find that this will impact your ability in a positive way to be more active, which, in turn, will help you to lose weight and feel younger. Imagine being able to play with your kids and grandkids without getting tired out as quickly as you had before. That is a benefit that will last and get better the longer that you participate in the DASH Diet.

Chapter 2: Helpful Tricks and Tips

Easy ways to get started today

Luckily, for the beginning participants of the DASH Diet, it is rather simple to start easily. The bottom line of the diet is to add more vegetables, fruits, and low-fat dairy products and to limit sugar, red meat, and, of course, sodium. You also want to include poultry, whole-grain, fish, and nuts into your cooking.

The best recommendation is to start cutting back your sodium levels gradually. Do not start at a daily goal of 1,500 mg of sodium, but rather about a teaspoon a day bringing the milligrams to 2,400.

This equates to approximately a teaspoon of salt a

day. It may sound like you are cutting back drastically, but I assure you that you will not taste the difference with the recipes I have in store for you.

After about a week on the diet, you can start to take your sodium numbers down towards the recommended levels of 1,500 mg. However, it is best to consult your physician because it depends on your personal activity level, ultimate goals, and health concerns at what level you personally need to hit each day. This is also inclusive of the number of calories you should be consuming.

A great tip to get started today is to go through your pantry, freezer, and fridge to remove the items that are high in salt, sugar, and fat. This includes processed foods as well.

Read the labels carefully as you might be surprised what can contain high levels of sodium. I recommend that you donate the items that you will no longer be eating to neighbors or to a local food bank so that it does not go to waste. You will also be helping out your community which will make you mentally feel great.

Once you rid yourself of the former tempting comfort foods, you will have plenty of room left for the more healthy choices that you can find in this cookbook. Your body will be thanking you for completing this task even though it may take a while.

You will find that many of these recipes can be cooked and stored ahead of time, making it quite easy to be able to stay on course with the DASH Diet. When you have healthy food choices easily accessible in your pantry and fridge, you will be less likely to go to the store around the corner to pick up your normal snacks.

Also, if you are going to be cooking for not just you but your family members as well, it can a bit tricky to make the transition. However, once they eat the nutritious meals and snacks you will be creating, they will also see the benefits themselves.

These recipes are easy enough to get the children and significant others in the kitchen teaching them healthier alternatives and getting to spend more quality time together as well.

Simple tips to make the shift today are to use only half of the condiments such as dressings and margarine that you are used to having on your meals. The recommended serving for margarine and dressings is a tablespoon which may take a bit getting used to with your possible former habits. However, this is a small yet significant change that will have large impacts on your overall health.

And since fruits and vegetables are going to be consumed more, stock up on these items and store them in your refrigerator and readily accessible on the countertop. Look for deals at your local farmer's market or grocery and look for the sale items to keep within your budget.

You can also use canned and frozen items but beware of any added salts or sugars that usually come with these varieties of food. Try to refrain from constantly eating dried fruits especially as they usually contain high amounts of sugar.

Snack time may have included junk foods in the past. A healthier alternative is to incorporate unsalted nuts, fat-free yogurt, or again fruits and vegetables.

Once you start making a habit of eating more nutritiously, it will be easier to stay on course with the DASH Diet.

Common Mistakes when Starting the Dash Diet

When you are faced with major medical issues, it is tempting to throw everything out that you have been doing before and jump in with enthusiasm. This is the mindset that you are going to need, but it is best to start slowly.

If you take baby steps into incorporating the changes in your life, they will more likely become the habits that will stay in place for some time to come. You will also find that when these healthy habits are formed, it will be easier to stay on track towards your goals as you will see the results that you crave.

As stated before, there are foods that have hidden sodium levels that you would not consider high since they are not overly salty tasting. However, it is most important to educate yourself on the foods that you have been eating that you may consider safe on the DASH Diet to make sure they will keep you within your personal daily limits.

As an example, many foods which are preserved contain higher amounts of salt, so close attention must be made to ensure you avoid these items. There are many alternatives to your favorite foods that you will find will be labeled with low-sodium. You will also find many of your favorites in this cookbook which have been converted to a healthier and better-tasting version. Mostly, it is about education and reading labels that will keep you on track.

Some people may not like the idea of cutting out the comfort foods they have enjoyed for quite some time. They may feel that if they just cut back to a smaller serving of these items, it is wise. This is a common mistake. It is best to find alternatives that satisfy your cravings that stay within the guidelines of the DASH Diet.

You will find if you follow the meal plan and recipes laid out in this cookbook that you will crave these items less. In fact, you may find that some of your comfort foods have been converted to a healthier recipe than you used before.

Keeping an eye on sugar levels also includes the beverages that you enjoy. Do not simply cut out fructose high soft drinks for fruit juices as these commonly have high amounts of added sugars as well.

Your morning cup of Joe is going to be a culprit for this scrutiny as well. Consider making black coffee at home with fat-free milk rather than getting a fancy coffee shop pick-me-up as they usually contain high amounts of sugar when combining flavors, creamers, and sweeteners.

Ways to be Successful

Set your personal goals for starting this diet and keep them somewhere visible. This could be on your bathroom mirror or on the fridge to constantly remind you why you are making this life change.

Maybe it could be a picture of how you want to look, a family picture, or even a dream vacation that you would like to take without the worries of your health. Anything that would keep you motivated towards your goals will keep your spirits up as you go through the changes the DASH Diet will bring to your life.

If it is a personal goal of yours to lose weight and you are not currently exercising, perhaps consider starting light by taking an evening walk, jog, or take a swimming course. Start small as you do not want to set yourself up for failure. This is also a good tip if you hit a plateau with your weight loss and that is one of your goals.

Another tip for weight loss is to limit the number of calories you are consuming. If you eat a smaller amount of calories than what you expend in a day, you will naturally lose those pounds.

Get the family on board with these changes in your relationship with food. Explain to them why it is necessary and they will be a fantastic support system for you and most likely take part in bettering yours and their health.

If you are doing this alone, find friends and groups that are doing the same diet. They will not only be a support system but a wealth of knowledge and experience, especially if they have been participants of the DASH Diet for a while.

Do not only change your relationship with food but your environment as well. You will not be able to just go to lunch with your co-workers, but you will have a healthy lunch that you have prepared ahead of time that you have brought with you. This will also help your pocketbook.

Some people go to the extreme and cut out salt altogether. This is a dangerous decision as it may have the opposite effect you desire. When you have too little sodium intake, it will put you at a higher risk of insulin resistance and heart disease, for instance.

The lowest amount that is recommended is approximately two-thirds of a teaspoon of salt a day. This will keep your body running at optimum level without the risk of harming yourself in the long run.

Take into account how much salt you are consuming now and gradually work your way down from that number. For instance, it may be that you have been eating about two teaspoons of salt. Consider lowering it to half at first and lower from there as required. Again, it is all about baby steps, and you will find the highest level of success.

This may seem like a lot to cut back your sodium intake by half. However, once you take out the processed foods, this will be easier than you think.

Again, you will be more successful when discussing your personal health goals with your healthcare professional who can advise you the most beneficial method in reaching your goals.

Chapter 3: Meal Program

There is a lot of variety that you can experience while on the DASH Diet so it will never get boring. This is because there is no particular checklist of foods you have to eat. Rather, you will be following a set amount of servings from each food group. Some simple tips to get an easy start to making your own meal plan are the following:

- 6 – 8 helpings of whole grains a day
  - Whole grain cereals, breads, oatmeal, quinoa, and pastas
- 4 – 5 helpings of vegetables a day
  - There are no vegetables that are limited in the DASH Diet and can be raw or cooked.
- 4 – 5 helpings of fruits a day
  - Berries, apples, mango, pineapple, pears, and peaches
- 2 – 3 helpings of dairy a day
  - You will want to have low-fat varieties such as yogurt, cheese, and skim

milk
- 6 ounces or fewer of meat and fish a day
    - You want to go with lean meats and you want to limit red meat consumption to two servings a week or less. This category also includes eggs.
- 2 – 3 helpings of oils and fats a day
    - Olive oil, mayonnaise, dressings, and margarine
- 4 – 5 helpings of legumes, seeds, and nuts a week.
    - Walnuts, peanuts, hazelnuts, almonds, lentils, beans, and peas.
- 5 helpings or less of sugars and candies
    - It is best to avoid this food group if possible to get the highest benefit from the DASH Diet. This includes granulated sugar, soda, and chocolates.
- Keep your salt levels between 1,500 mg and 2,300 mg a day.
- Coffee and alcohol can be consumed, but know that this also raises blood pressure levels and puts you more at risk for heart disease. Refrain from having more than a beverage in twenty-four hours for women with two

beverages daily for men.

Still a little overwhelming? No worries! Here is a Sample Menu for your first week on the DASH Diet. Feel free to mix and match the days as you desire. That is the beauty of the diet as you are free to make your own food choices as long as you stay within the serving guidelines. Every item that is in italics are recipes that can be found in this cookbook and focuses on the typical 2,000 calorie-a-day diet.

Weekly Sample Menu

Monday

Breakfast

- One slice of whole wheat bread with a teaspoon of margarine
- One helping of *Creamy Oatmeal* (pg 51)
- One apple
- One cup milk, low-fat or skim
- Decaffeinated coffee

Lunch

- One helping of *Quinoa Salad* with a tablespoon of *Yogurt Dressing*
- 12 low-sodium crackers, whole wheat
- One banana
- One cup milk, low-fat or skim
- Water

Snack

- One cup *Trail Mix*
- One cup of fat-free yogurt

Dinner

- One helping *Cauliflower Rice* (pg 266)
- 4 ounces lean chicken
- One cup of steamed broccoli & carrot mix
- Herbal Tea
- Water

Tuesday

Breakfast

- Two *Oatmeal Pancakes* (pg 67) with One tablespoon of maple syrup or One-fourth cup berries
- One tablespoon margarine
- 4 oz. orange juice, no added sugars
- One peach
- Decaffeinated coffee

Lunch

- One *Chicken Gyro* with One tablespoon of *Tzatziki Sauce*
- One cup of mixed fruit such as mango and pineapple or apples and bananas
- One helping of *Stuffed Mushrooms*
- Water

Snack

- One-fourth cup of celery with two tablespoons *Peanut Butter,* low-sodium
- One medium orange
- One helping of *Apple Crumb Cake Muffins* (pg 260)
- Herbal tea

Dinner

- One helping of *Pumpkin Soup* with One-half cup of walnuts or peanuts, unsalted
- 12 crackers, whole wheat
- One helping of *Zucchini Frittata* with One tablespoon of *Ranch Dressing*
- One iced herbal tea

Wednesday

Breakfast

- One helping of *Stuffed Potatoes* (pg 72) with One tablespoon of margarine
- One cup of skim milk
- One-half cup of mixed berries
- Decaffeinated coffee

Lunch

- One helping of *Fettuccine Alfredo* (pg 100)
- One cup of *Herbed Oven Roasted Veggies*
- One-half cup of cherry tomatoes
- Water

Snack

- One helping of *Fiesta Dip*
- 12 crackers, whole wheat
- One pear

Dinner

- One helping of *Baked Salmon* with One tablespoon of *Tartar Sauce*
- One helping of *Carrot Dip*
- One cup of yogurt, fat-free
- One-half cup of blueberries
- Water
- Herbal Tea

Thursday

Breakfast

- One helping of *Eggs Benedict*
- One helping of *Homemade Bacon*
- One piece of toast, whole wheat with One tablespoon of margarine
- One-half cup raspberries with 8 ounces of Greek yogurt, low-fat
- One-half cup orange juice, no sugar added

Lunch

- One helping of *Mexican Salad*
- One helping of *South American Guacamole*
- One-half cup cucumbers, sliced
- Water
- One-half cup pineapple

Snack

- One helping *Peanut Butter Bar*

- One cup milk, skim
- 4 ounces of blackberries

Dinner

- One helping of *Red Pepper Hummus*
- One helping of *Red Beans & Rice*
- One-half cup broccoli, steamed
- One-half cup of green peas

Friday

Breakfast

- One cup of low-fat yogurt
- One helping of *Biscuits & Gravy*
- One cup skim milk
- One cup mix of strawberries and

blueberries
- Decaffeinated coffee

Lunch

- One helping *Turkey Panini* topped with lettuce, tomato, and one tablespoon of *Mayonnaise*
- One helping of *Mozzarella Sticks* with One tablespoon of marinara sauce
- One helping of *Fried Rice*
- Water

Snack

- Two tablespoons of *Peanut Butter*, low-sodium on One medium banana
- One cup of fat-free yogurt

Dinner

- One helping of *Vegetarian Chili* with One tablespoon of sour cream, low-fat
- One helping of *Macaroni & Cheese* (pg 273)
- One cup of brown rice
- 12 whole wheat crackers
- Herbal Tea

Saturday

Breakfast

- One helping of *Breakfast Tostadas* with one tablespoon of sour cream, low-fat
- One helping of *Sausage Patties*
- One helping *Green Smoothie*
- One medium banana
- One-half cup of Greek Yogurt
- Herbal Tea

Lunch

- One helping of *Crunchy Fried Chicken*
- One helping of *Mashed Potatoes* with three teaspoons of margarine or three teaspoons of low-fat sour cream
- One boiled egg

- One-half cup applesauce, no sugar added
- Water

Snack

- One-half cup almonds, unsalted
- One cup fruit salad

Dinner

- One helping *Veggie Lasagna*
- One helping *Zesty Mushroom Soup*
- One whole wheat roll with one tablespoon of margarine
- Iced herbal tea

Sunday

Breakfast

- One helping of *Bacon Egg & Spinach Casserole*
- One *Fruit Smoothie*
- One slice whole wheat toast with one tablespoon of fruit jam, no sugar added
- One cup skim milk
- Decaffeinated coffee

Lunch

- One helping *Sloppy Joes*
- One helping *Potato Salad*
- One medium banana
- One helping of *Lintel Stew*
- Water
- Iced herbal tea

Snack

- One-half cup low-fat chocolate pudding
- Two tablespoons of low-sodium *Peanut Butter* on one medium banana

Dinner

- One helping of *Black Bean Burgers* with one tablespoon of *Mustard, Ketchup,* and *Mayonnaise*
- One helping of *Minestrone Soup*
- One-half cup tomatoes, two cups mixed greens topped with one tablespoon of *Avocado Dressing*
- Herbal Tea

Nutritional Information Note for this Cookbook

Nutritional information for the recipes provided is an approximate only. And substitutions that you use will alter the nutritional values and need to be personally researched to define the true macronutrients. As such, we cannot guarantee the complete accuracy of the nutritional information given for any recipe in this cookbook. The macronutrients are calculated by one helping size and for what is included in the ingredients listing.

Chapter 4: Breakfast Recipes

Bacon Egg & Spinach Casserole

Total Prep & Cooking Time: 55 minutes

Makes: 4 Helpings

Sodium: 365 mg

Protein: 20 gm

Fat: 10 gm

Sugar: 2 gm

Calories: 173

What you need:

- One-fourth tsp. black pepper
- One-third green bell pepper, chopped
- Twenty-four oz. spinach
- Three-fourths cup cheddar, shredded
- One cup egg whites

- Two-thirds cup mushrooms, sliced
- 4 slices bacon, low-sodium (See Helpful Tip below)
- Two tbsp. olive oil, separated
- One-third cup red onion, chopped
- olive oil cooking spray
- One-fourth tsp. salt
- One large egg
- One-third red bell pepper, chopped

Steps:

1. Scrub the bell pepper and mushrooms thoroughly. Chop the bell pepper and slice the mushrooms and set to the side.
2. Remove the outer skin from the onion and chop into small sections. Set to the side.
3. Empty one tablespoon of the oil into a pan and arrange the sliced bacon so they are not touching. Brown for approximately two minutes

while flipping over as needed to fry to your preferred crispiness.

4. Transfer to a platter layered with kitchen paper and set to the side to cool.

5. Adjust your stove to heat at the temperature of 375° Fahrenheit. Apply olive oil to a glass baking dish and set to the side.

6. Transfer the 3hree teaspoons of oil that remains into the skillet and combine the chopped mushrooms, onion, and bell pepper into the pan.

7. Heat for approximately three minutes. Half of the vegetables should be distributed using a slotted spoon on the prepped baking dish' base.

8. Layer the spinach over the vegetables and empty the remaining cooked vegetables on top of the spinach.

9. Use a glass dish to combine the pepper, egg, egg whites, and salt until integrated. Empty the dish on top of the cooked vegetables.

10. Take the cooked bacon and crush into small chunks over the eggs and dust with the shredded cheese.

11. Heat in the stove for 35 minutes and remove to the counter.

12. Wait about a quarter of an hour before serving and enjoy!

Helpful Tip:

- You can use the recipe for *homemade bacon* which can be found in this chapter.

Biscuits & Gravy

Total Prep & Cooking Time: 5 minutes

Makes: 1 Smoothie

Sodium: 24 mg

Protein: 8 gm

Fat: 7 gm

Sugar: 6 gm

Calories: 272

What you need:

- One and one-fourth cups whole wheat flour, separated
- One-half tsp. Mrs. Dash's Table Blend, salt-free
- Two tbsp. olive oil
- One-fourth tsp. black pepper
- One oz. margarine
- One-half tbsp. baking powder, salt-free

- One-half tsp. sugar, granulated
- One-fourth tsp. salt
- One and one-half cup milk, skim and separated

Steps:

1. Adjust the stove temperature to heat at 425° Fahrenheit. Layer a flat sheet with baking lining and set to the side.
2. Use a glass dish to blend the baking powder, one cup of the flour, seasoning, margarine, and granulated sugar until there is no more lumpiness present.
3. Finally, integrate 8 ounces of the milk to the mixture and blend until it becomes thick dough.
4. Dust a flat surface with 2 tablespoons of the flour and flatten the pastry to be about one-inch thick.
5. Use a glass or a cookie cutter that is at least 2 inches in diameter, cut the dough into 6 individual circles.
6. Arrange on the prepped flat sheet and

heat for approximately 14 minutes.

7. In the meantime, heat the olive oil, pepper, leftover 1/8 cup of flour, the leftover one-half cup of the skim milk, and salt in a skillet.

8. Warm gently for about 10 minutes as the gravy reduces while occasionally stirring.

9. Transfer the biscuits from the stove and move onto individual serving plates.

10. Slice them in half and drizzle the gravy over the top.

11. Serve immediately and enjoy!

Breakfast Tostadas

Total Prep & Cooking Time: 30 minutes

Makes: 4 Helpings

Sodium: 270 mg

Protein: 20 gm

Fat: 22 gm

Sugar: 5 gm

Calories: 371

What you need:

- 8 corn tortillas, low-sodium
- Two scallions, sliced thinly
- 8 tbsp. cream cheese, low-fat
- One tsp. Tabasco hot sauce
- Two small tomatoes, deseeded and chopped
- One medium jalapeno, chopped
- 8 large eggs

- Two slices Swiss cheese, low-sodium
- Three tbsp. cilantro, chopped
- olive oil cooking spray

Steps:

1. Set your stove to the temperature of 375° Fahrenheit.
2. Place the jalapeno pepper over the stove burner on the setting of a medium.
3. Use a pair of tongs to flip the pepper over as it begins to turn black. This should take approximately two minutes.
4. Turn the burner off and move the jalapeno with the tongs to a paper towel for about 5 minutes.
5. In the meantime, arrange the tortillas onto to the rack in the stove so they will not fall through.
6. Heat for approximately 6 minutes and remove carefully to serving dishes.
7. Put on a pair of gloves and rub the skin off of the jalapeno and chop finely. Set to the side.
8. Thoroughly wash the tomatoes and chop

the scallions and tomatoes. Set aside.

9. Blend the cream cheese and Tabasco sauce in a glass dish until the consistency is smooth. Set to the side.

10. Coat a pan with the oil spray and heat the chopped jalapeno for about 90 seconds.

11. In a separate dish, whip the eggs and transfer the chopped scallions into the dish.

12. Empty the eggs into the skillet and stir occasionally allowing the eggs to set for approximately 60 seconds.

13. Combine the chopped tomatoes and sliced cheese to the skillet and heat for another 2 minutes. Remove from the burner.

14. Evenly distribute the sour cream to each tortilla, spreading almost to the edges.

15. Divide the egg mixture evenly between each of the tortillas and serve immediately.

Creamy Oatmeal

Total Prep & Cooking Time: 10 minutes

Makes: 4 Helpings

Sodium: 7 mg

Protein: 18 gm

Fat: 21 gm

Sugar: 12 gm

Calories: 568

What you need:

- One cup of berries of choice
- Two cups oats, old fashioned
- One and one-third cup almonds, sliced
- Three and one-fourth cups water
- One tbsp. ground cinnamon
- Two medium bananas

Steps:

1. Crush the bananas thoroughly until smooth.
2. Empty the water into a saucepan and incorporate the mashed banana.
3. Combine the oats in the pan and heat until the water bubbles.
4. Adjust the temperature of the burner to low and continue to warm for approximately 7 minutes.
5. Remove from heat and top with the ground cinnamon, berries, and sliced almonds.
6. Serve immediately and enjoy!

Helpful Tip:

- There are many options of toppings you can use to add variety to this meal. Some options are granola, maple syrup, honey, or brown sugar.

Egg Salad

Total Prep& Cooking Time: 15 minutes

Makes: One Salad

Sodium: 309 mg

Protein: 22 gm

Fat: 21 gm

Sugar: 6 gm

Calories: 314

What you need:

- One and one-half cups pre-packaged salad greens
- One/eight cup mozzarella cheese
- One cup sweet bell pepper of your choice, chopped
- One-fourth tsp. black pepper
- One tbsp. avocado, diced
- Two large eggs

- Three-fourths cup tomato, chopped
- One-fourth tsp. salt
- eight cups cold water, separated
- One tsp. thyme, crushed
- One-half cup cucumber, sliced
- One tsp. olive oil

Steps:

1. Empty 4 cups of the cold water into a stockpot with the eggs and turn the burner on.
2. When the water starts to bubble, set a timer for 7 minutes.
3. Meanwhile, scrub and chop the tomato, cucumber, avocado, and bell pepper and transfer to a salad dish.
4. After the timer has chimed, remove the hot water and empty the remaining 4 cups of cold water on top of the eggs. Set aside for approximately 5 minutes.
5. Once the eggs have cooled, peel the shell and dice into small sections and transfer to the dish.
6. Combine the salad greens and shredded

mozzarella cheese to the salad dish and turn until integrated with the vegetables.

7. Dispense the olive oil over the dish and blend the crushed thyme, pepper, and salt until mixed well.

8. Serve immediately and enjoy!

Eggs Benedict

Total Prep & Cooking Time: 15 minutes

Makes: Two Helpings

Sodium: 502 mg

Protein: 15 gm

Fat: 8 gm

Sugar: 5 gm

Calories: 201

What you need:

- One-half cup water
- Two tomato slices
- Three tbsp. sour cream, fat-free
- One whole wheat English muffin, low-sodium
- Two tsp. milk, fat-free
- One tsp. mustard, low-sodium (See Helpful Tip below)

- Two large eggs
- One tbsp. chives, chopped
- Two oz. ham slices, low-sodium
- olive oil cooking spray

Steps:

1. Adjust the stove temperature to broil. Prepare a flat sheet with a section of tin foil to use later.

2. Blend the sour cream, mustard, and milk in a glass dish and set to the side.

3. Slice the English muffin into two and set on the prepped flat sheet.

4. Heat in the stove for about two minutes.

5. In the meantime, use olive oil to coat a pan and then pour in the water.

6. Heat until it bubbles and then turn the burner down to low.

7. Open one of the eggs and put into an additional glass dish.

8. Slowly distribute the full egg to the simmering water, trying not to break the

yolk.

9. Repeat steps 7 and 8 for the other egg and make sure they are not touching. Warm for about 4 minutes.

10. Withdraw the muffins from the stove and layer the ham and tomato evenly on each of the muffins and broil for another 60 seconds.

11. Transfer the eggs with a spoon with holes and transfer to the prepared muffins.

12. Distribute the topping over the eggs liberally and dust with the chopped chives.

13. Serve immediately and enjoy!

Helpful Tip:

- You can find a healthy low-sodium mustard recipe in Chapter 7.

Fruit Smoothie

Total Prep & Cooking Time: 5 minutes

Makes: One Smoothie

Sodium: 71e mg

Protein: 6 gm

Fat: 3 gm

Sugar: 26 gm

Calories: 184

What you need:

- One-fourth cup blueberries
- Four oz. strawberries
- One-half orange, peeled
- Four oz. papaya peeled, seeded and diced
- One-fourth cup ice cubes
- Four oz. soy milk

Steps:

1. Pulse the blueberries, strawberries, peeled orange, and milk in a blender for approximately half a minute.
2. Combine the ice cubes and papaya and continue to blend for another 30 seconds.
3. Transfer to a glass and enjoy immediately.

Helpful Tips:

- Get creative with this recipe by adding in a quarter cup of ground flax seeds, chia seeds, or banana.

- You can also use frozen fruit if you prefer.

Green Smoothie

Total Prep & Cooking Time: 5 minutes

Makes: One Smoothie

Sodium: 20 mg

Protein: 2 gm

Fat: 0 gm

Sugar: 5 gm

Calories: 48

What you need:

- One-fourth cup yogurt, non-fat and plain
- One-half tsp. vanilla extract
- One cup spinach
- One medium banana
- One-half cup milk, fat-free
- Three-fourths cup mango
- One-fourth cup whole oats

Steps:

1. Using a blender, combine the baby spinach, yogurt, whole oats, milk, and mango. Pulse for approximately half a minute.

2. Blend the banana and vanilla extract and pulse for an additional half minute until smooth.

3. Empty into a serving glass and enjoy immediately.

Homemade Bacon

Total Prep & Cooking Time: 80 minutes

Makes: 4 Helpings

Sodium: 122 mg

Protein: 4 gm

Fat: 24 gm

Sugar: 4 gm

Calories: 253

What you need:

- One tsp. cumin seasoning
- One tsp. black pepper
- Two tbsp. olive oil
- Sixteen oz. pork belly, sliced no more than one-fourth inch thick
- Four tsp. liquid smoke
- Two tsp. smoked paprika seasoning
- Three tbsp. maple syrup

- One-fourth tsp. salt

Steps:

1. Set your stove to the temperature of 200° Fahrenheit. Cover a flat sheet with a rim with foil. Set to the side.
2. Remove the rind from the pork belly slices by using kitchen scissors and arrange the slices on the prepped baking pan so they are in a single layer and not touching.
3. Utilize another pan if necessary depending on the thickness of your bacon.
4. In a glass dish, blend the maple syrup and the liquid smoke until integrated.
5. In a separate dish, combine the pepper, cumin, and smoked paprika fully.
6. Use a pastry brush to apply the maple syrup to each of the bacon slices.
7. Turn the slices over and repeat step 5.
8. Dust all of the slices with the mixed seasonings and rub the spices into the meat.
9. Heat in the stove for 60 minutes and remove.

10. The bacon is ready to be stored or fried. See the Helpful Tips below for storing instructions.

11. Empty the olive oil into a skillet and arrange the slices in a single layer. You will need to cook in stages.

12. Brown for approximately two minutes while turning over as needed to fully fry to your desired crispiness.

13. Remove to a paper towel covered plate and enjoy while hot!

Helpful Tips:

- If you have thicker cut pork belly slices, you will only need one pan for this recipe. If you have the thinner cut slices, you will need to use two. They can be placed in the oven at the same time.

- To store the pre-cooked bacon, set in a

lidded tub for 5 days in the fridge.

- If freezing, wrap in freezer or wax paper in between the slices and store for three months. Allow to defrost in the fridge at least 6 hours before frying.

Oatmeal Pancakes

Total Prep & Cooking Time: 30 minutes

Makes: 4 Pancakes

Sodium: 116 mg

Protein: 9 gm

Fat: 3 gm

Sugar: 6 gm

Calories: 150

What you need:

- One-half tsp. ground cinnamon
- 4 oz. whole wheat flour
- Two oz. oats, old fashioned
- One tsp. baking powder, salt-free
- One/eight tsp. salt
- olive oil cooking spray
- 4 oz. milk, skim
- One/eight cup Greek yogurt, no-fat

- One large egg
- One-half tsp. vanilla extract
- Three tsp. brown sugar

Steps:

1. In a big dish, blend the salt, whole wheat flour, ground cinnamon, whole oats, and baking powder combining completely.
2. Using another dish, fully integrate the milk and egg until the mixed well.
3. Combine the vanilla extract, yogurt, and brown sugar into the eggs and whisk to remove any lumpiness.
4. Slowly empty the egg dish into the flour dish making sure it is totally combined but do not mix too thoroughly.
5. Warm a skillet. Make sure the skillet is sprayed with olive oil.
6. Distribute approximately a quarter of the batter into the skillet.
7. Turn the pancake over after the top starts to bubble after about 60 seconds.
8. Let the pancake cook for approximately

another minute and flip as needed until browned completely.

9. Remove to a plate and coat the skillet with an additional coat of olive oil spray.

10. Perform steps 6 through 9 until all the pancakes are finished.

11. Serve while hot and enjoy!

Helpful Tip:

- If you would like to be creative with this recipe, combine one-fourth cup of fruit into the batter before transferring to the hot skillet. Of course, you can add your fruits on top before serving.

Sausage Patties

Total Prep & Cooking Time: 15 minutes

Makes: 4 Helpings

Sodium: 36 mg

Protein: 10 gm

Fat: 11 gm

Sugar: 0 gm

Calories: 148

What you need:

- One-half tsp. black pepper
- Eight oz. pork, ground and lean
- olive oil cooking spray
- One-half tsp. thyme seasoning
- Two tbsp. chicken broth, low-salt (See Helpful Tip below)
- One-half tsp. red pepper flakes
- One-fourth tsp. sage seasoning

Steps:

1. Set a foot-long section of wax paper onto the counter.
2. In a big glass dish, blend the pepper, sage, pork, thyme, chicken broth, and red pepper flakes by hand until fully incorporated.
3. Equally divide the meat into 8 individual mounds and arrange on the left side of the wax paper.
4. Fold the wax paper to cover the patties and flatten to the desired thickness.
5. Apply a coat of oil spray to a pan and brown the meat for about 5 minutes.
6. Turn the patties to the other side and fry for an additional 5 minutes.
7. Distribute to the individual platters and enjoy immediately.

Helpful Tip:

- There is a healthy low-sodium chicken broth recipe located in Chapter 7.

Stuffed Potatoes

Total Prep & Cooking Time: 45 minutes

Makes: 4 Helpings

Sodium: 234 mg

Protein: 10 gm

Fat: 1 gm

Sugar: 1 gm

Calories: 198

What you need:

- One-third cup red bell pepper, chopped finely
- One/eight tsp. black pepper
- Sixteen oz. russet potatoes
- One-third cup Mexican cheese blend,

shredded

- One/eight tsp. salt
- One-fourth cup scallions, sliced
- Two tbsp. margarine
- Three large eggs

Steps:

1. Poke the potatoes about 5 times with a fork and nuke for 5 minutes in the microwave.

2. Use oven mitts to flip the potatoes over and heat for another 4 minutes.

3. Take out from the microwave with oven mitts and wait for approximately 10 minutes to cool.

4. In the meantime, prepare the scallions and the bell pepper by thoroughly scrubbing. Slice the scallions and chop the bell pepper and set to the side.

5. Divide the potatoes in two and take out the insides of the potato, leaving approximately a quarter inch at the skins.

6. Adjust the temperature of your stove to 425° Fahrenheit. Cover a flat sheet with baking

lining or foil and set to the side.

7. Dissolve the margarine in a skillet and combine the potato meat, scallions, and bell pepper.

8. Heat for about 4 minutes while tossing often.

9. Combine the pepper, eggs, and salt into the pan and warm for another two minutes. Turn the burner off and blend the cheese fully into the filling.

10. Scoop the filling into each of the potato skins and set them on the prepped baking sheet.

11. Wait for about 5 minutes before enfolding the entire potato in foil and arrange back on the flat pan.

12. Heat in the stove for approximately eighteen minutes and carefully remove.

13. Take the foil off the potatoes and enjoy immediately.

Quiche Cups

Total Prep & Cooking Time: 45 minutes

Makes: 4 Helpings

Sodium: 64 mg

Protein: 6 gm

Fat: 6 gm

Sugar: 2 gm

Calories: 89

What you need:

- One-half scallion, diced finely
- Five oz. broccoli, frozen and chopped
- One-fourth cup bell pepper of your choice, diced finely
- Two large eggs
- One-half tsp. hot sauce
- Three-eight cup ricotta cheese, skim milk
- One-fourth tsp. black pepper

Steps:

1. Nuke the broccoli in the microwave for about two minutes until completely thawed.
2. Remove and use a clean dish towel to wring the excess moisture out of the broccoli and set to the side.
3. Arrange 4 silicon or paper baking cups in a cupcake tin and set your stove to heat at the temperature of 350° Fahrenheit.
4. Wash the bell peppers and the scallion well and dice into small sections. Set to the side and transfer to a glass dish.
5. Combine the broccoli, eggs, hot sauce, ricotta cheese, and pepper into the dish and blend until incorporated fully.
6. Evenly distribute the batter to the baking cups.
7. Heat the cupcake tin for half an hour and remove to a wire rack.
8. Wait for about 5 minutes before serving and enjoy!

Helpful Tip:

- You can use any other frozen vegetable you would like in place of the broccoli if you prefer to add variety to this recipe.

Chapter 5: Lunch Recipes

American Chopsuey

Total Prep & Cooking Time: 30 minutes

Makes: 4 Helpings

Sodium: 557 mg

Protein: 28 gm

Fat: 17 gm

Sugar: 3 gm

Calories: 512

What you need:

- Two tsp. olive oil
- Twelve oz. beef, ground
- Two tsp. paprika seasoning
- One cup bell pepper, color of your choice and chopped

- Two-thirds tsp. black pepper
- One One-third cups tomato, diced
- Two One-half cloves garlic, diced
- 11 oz. canned tomato sauce, salt-free (See Helpful Tip below)
- Two-thirds tbsp. vinegar, red wine
- 12 oz. elbow macaroni, whole wheat
- Two-thirds cup onion, chopped
- 6 oz. Swiss cheese, shredded
- Sixteen cups water
- One-fourth tsp. salt

Steps:

1. Thoroughly wash the bell pepper and tomato and slice into small cubes.

2. Remove the outer layer of the onion and dice into small sections.

3. Empty the water into a deep pot with the elbow macaroni and the salt. Heat for about 10 minutes.

4. Meanwhile, using a skillet and for thirty seconds, heat the olive oil and combine the chopped bell pepper and onion, garlic, and

ground beef.

5. Use a wooden spatula to continue to break apart the meat and fry for approximately 8 minutes.

6. Blend the tomato sauce, chopped tomatoes, pepper, red wine vinegar, and paprika until incorporated and bring to a rumbling boil for approximately 10 minutes, occasionally agitating.

7. Separate the water from the noodles and blend in the skillet, fully coating with the sauce.

8. Serve immediately and enjoy!

Helpful Tip:

- You can use the healthy low-sodium marinara sauce recipe in place of the tomato paste. It is found in Chapter 7.

Asian Chicken Wraps

Total Prep & Cooking Time: 30 minutes

Makes: 4 Wraps

Sodium: 534 mg

Protein: 27 gm

Fat: 22 gm

Sugar: 10 gm

Calories: 364

What you need:

For the chicken:

- Four scallions, chopped
- One oz. carrot, chopped
- Four oz. peanuts, unsalted
- One cup red bell pepper, chopped
- Four Romaine lettuce heart leaves

- Sixteen oz. chicken, ground
- Four cloves garlic, minced
- One tbsp. olive oil

For the sauce:

- Three tbsp. soy sauce, low-sodium (See Helpful Tip below)
- One-half tbsp. lemon juice
- One-half tbsp. ginger powder
- Three tbsp. brown sugar

Steps:

1. In a glass dish, blend the lemon juice, soy sauce, ginger powder, and brown sugar, whisking to ensure there is no lumpiness present. Set to the side.
2. Warm up the olive oil in a pan for about 30

seconds and transfer the ground chicken to the pan.

3. Fry for approximately 10 minutes while breaking into smaller chunks with a wooden spatula.

4. Prepare the scallions, carrot, and bell pepper by scrubbing thoroughly and chopping into small sections.

5. Transfer the chopped vegetables and the garlic into the pan and heat for an additional 5 minutes.

6. Lay out the individual lettuce leaves onto a serving platter.

7. Empty the sauce from the glass dish into the skillet and cover the meat completely.

8. Ladle the filling evenly into the each of the lettuce leaves.

9. Sprinkle the peanuts on top of the lettuce leaves and enjoy immediately.

Helpful Tip:

- There is a recipe for a healthy low-sodium version of soy sauce in Chapter 7.

Baked Chicken

Total Prep & Cooking Time: 30 minutes

Makes: 4 Helpings

Sodium: 403 mg

Protein: 46 gm

Fat: 7 gm

Sugar: 4 gm

Calories: 286

What you need:

For the chicken:

- 4 chicken breasts, no bones or skins
- Two tsp. olive oil

For the seasoning:

- One-half tsp. black pepper
- One and one-half tbsp. brown sugar
- One tsp. thyme seasoning
- One tsp. paprika seasoning
- One-half tsp. salt
- One-fourth tsp. garlic powder

For the garnish:

- One tbsp. parsley, chopped

Steps:

1. Heat the stove to the temperature of 425°

Fahrenheit. Prepare a flat sheet with a rim with a layer of foil and set to the side.

2. Blend the paprika, brown sugar, thyme, pepper, garlic powder, and salt in a glass dish until combined.

3. Arrange the chicken upside down on the prepped flat sheet and apply one tablespoon of the olive oil with a pastry brush.

4. Dust with half of the mixed seasoning, covering completely and turn the chicken to the other side.

5. Apply the remaining tablespoon of olive oil and the remaining seasoning making sure the chicken is completely covered.

6. Heat for 18 minutes and remove from the stove.

7. Wait about 5 minutes before enjoying immediately.

Helpful Tip:

- For variety, this recipe will go well with the low-sodium barbeque sauce found in Chapter 7. Simply brush the chicken with a brush to distribute the sauce after the seasonings and cook as instructed.

- You want to make sure that your chicken is about one-half inch thick for this recipe.

Cheesy Mushroom Risotto

Total Prep & Cooking Time: 30 minutes

Makes: 4 Helpings

Sodium: 123 mg

Protein: 20 gm

Fat: 8 gm

Sugar: 5 gm

Calories: 468

What you need:

- One and three-fourths cups Swiss cheese, finely grated
- One medium onion, peeled and chopped
- Two tbsp. water
- Four and one-half cups vegetable broth, low-salt (See Helpful Tip below)
- Two tbsp. lemon juice
- One-fourth cup white wine

- Two cups brown rice, uncooked
- One-third cup peas, thawed
- Two tbsp. olive oil, separated
- One-fourth tsp. black pepper
- One large leek, sliced thinly
- One and one-third cups mushrooms, sliced

Steps:

1. Remove the skin of the onion and chop into small chunks. Set to the side.
2. Wipe any excess dirt off of the mushrooms, slice and set aside.
3. Empty the vegetable broth into a deep pot and heat for approximately three minutes until it starts to bubble.
4. In the meantime, drizzle one tablespoon in a shallow skillet and brown the leeks, onion and two tablespoons of water for about two minutes.
5. Combine the rice, lemon juice, wine, and a cup of the vegetable stock.
6. Reduce while simmering for approximately

10 minutes until the water has completely evaporated.

7. Blend the mushrooms and add another cup of the vegetable stock, allowing to reduce completely.

8. Keep adding a cup of vegetable stock as the water evaporates completely until it has been fully used. This will take about half an hour.

9. Finally, blend the Swiss cheese and peas to the stockpot and heat for another three minutes.

10. Serve immediately and enjoy!

Helpful Tip:

- In Chapter 7, you will find the healthy alternative low-sodium recipe for vegetable broth.

Chicken Gyros

Total Prep & Cooking Time: 10 minutes

Makes: 4 Helpings

Sodium: 388 mg

Protein: 4 gm

Fat: 5 gm

Sugar: 2 gm

Calories: 159

What you need:

- Two tbsp. lemon juice
- One tsp. cumin seasoning
- 4 pita bread slices
- One-half tsp. paprika seasoning
- One-fourth tsp. salt
- Two tsp. oregano seasoning
- One tsp. rosemary seasoning
- One-half cup onion, sliced

- 4 tbsp. olive oil
- One-half cup scallion, sliced
- Two cloves garlic, minced
- Two lb. chicken breast, no bones or skins
- One-fourth tsp. black pepper

Steps:

1. Prepare the onion by removing the outer skin and slicing along with the scallion. Set to the side.
2. Slice the chicken breast into small strips and transfer to a glass dish.
3. Heat a skillet on the burner.
4. Blend the paprika, cumin, lemon juice, salt, olive oil, and minced garlic in the dish with the chicken until integrated.
5. Finally, combine the oregano, rosemary, and pepper into the chicken dish.
6. Toss to ensure the chicken is evenly coated and transfer to the hot pan.
7. Heat for approximately 6 minutes while

occasionally turning the meat to brown evenly.

8. Meanwhile, lay out the pita breads and top with the onions and green peppers.

9. Distribute the cooked chicken slices evenly on each of the pita breads.

10. Rotate the bread around the filling and enjoy immediately.

Helpful Tips:

- If you would like to have Tzatziki sauce on your gyro, you can find a healthy recipe in Chapter 7.

- You can also add chopped cucumbers or pickles to liven up this recipe.

Chicken Salad

Total Prep & Cooking Time: 25 minutes

Makes: 4 Helpings

Sodium: 272 mg

Protein: 18 gm

Fat: 10 gm

Sugar: 3 gm

Calories: 189

What you need:

- One large egg
- One-fourth tsp. salt
- One6 oz. canned chicken, low-sodium
- One/eight tsp. black pepper
- Three tbsp. red onion, chopped finely
- One-third cup mayonnaise, low-fat (See Helpful Tips below)
- Two tbsp. celery, chopped finely

- One tbsp. pickle relish
- 4 cups cold water

Steps:

1. Transfer half of the cold water into a pot to cover the egg.
2. Adjust a timer for 7 minutes as the water starts to bubble.
3. In the meantime, scrub and chop the red onion and celery into small sections. Set to the side.
4. After the timer has passed, remove the hot water and empty the remaining two cups of cold water on top of the egg. Set to the side.
5. Once the egg is easy to handle, remove the shell and dice into small cubes. Transfer to a glass dish.
6. Combine the onion, celery, and chicken with the egg and integrate well.
7. Use another glass dish to blend the salt, mayonnaise, relish, and pepper completely.
8. Empty the mayonnaise into the chicken and incorporate fully. If the mixture is too dry,

add another tablespoon of mayonnaise until the desired consistency.

9. Immediately serve and enjoy!

Helpful Tips:

- To add variety to this recipe, you can substitute different pickles of your choice for the relish such as bread and butter or dill pickles.

- There is a healthy low-sodium recipe for mayonnaise in Chapter 7.

Fettuccine Alfredo

Total Prep & Cooking Time: 30 minutes

Makes: 4 Helpings

Sodium: 363 mg

Protein: 28 gm

Fat: 18 gm

Sugar: 5 gm

Calories: 565

What you need:

- 6 oz. mozzarella cheese, shredded
- One and one-half cups milk, skim
- 6 cups water
- Two tbsp. olive oil
- One-fourth tsp. red pepper flakes
- One tsp. parsley seasoning
- 4 oz. Parmesan cheese, grated
- One tsp. basil seasoning

- Two oz. whole wheat flour
- One-half tsp. salt, separated
- 4 cloves garlic, minced
- One tsp. onion powder
- One6 oz. fettuccine noodles, whole wheat
- One-fourth tsp. black pepper
- One and one-half cups chicken broth, low-salt (See Helpful Tip below)

Steps:

1. Prepare the fettuccine noodles as required on the packaging using the 6 cups of water to bubble in a deep pot along with one-fourth teaspoon of the salt.

2. Meanwhile, warm the olive oil and garlic in a skillet for about 60 seconds.

3. Empty the flour into the pan and heat for approximately 4 minutes while continuously stirring.

4. Turn the heat to the lowest setting.
5. Use a metal whisk to combine the milk and the chicken broth making sure to stir non-stop.
6. Adjust the temperature to medium and bring the non-stick pan to a slow bubble.
7. Remove the fettuccine from the heat before the next steps.
8. Blend the red pepper flakes, onion powder, salt, basil, parsley, and pepper while continuing to stir.
9. Allow to reduce for approximately 5 minutes while stirring every once in a while.
10. Set the temperature to low once again and blend the parmesan and mozzarella cheese for about half a minute. Remove from the burner.
11. Separate the water from the fettuccine noodles and distribute to the pan with the alfredo sauce. Cover the noodles completely in the sauce and serve while hot.

Helpful Tip:

- Find the alternative low-sodium healthy version of the chicken broth recipe in Chapter 7.

Fish Fillets

Total Prep & Cooking Time: 15 minutes

Makes: 4 Helpings

Sodium: 380 mg

Protein: 36 gm

Fat: 16 gm

Sugar: 0 gm

Calories: 396

What you need:

- One and one-half tsp. Old Bay seasoning, salt-free
- Sixteen oz. cod fillet, thawed
- Three/eight cup canned light coconut milk
- 6 tbsp. white rice flour
- Three tbsp. olive oil

Steps:

1. Empty the coconut milk into a glass dish.
2. Use another dish to blend the Old Bay seasoning and the flour until combined.
3. Divide the cod into 4 equal sections and make sure all the moisture is removed.
4. Use a skillet to warm the olive oil.
5. Coat one piece of fish fully in the flour and immerse in the milk making sure all extra batter is removed.
6. Return the fish to the flour dish and completely cover.
7. Transfer the battered cod to the hot skillet and heat for approximately three minutes before flipping to the other side for another two minutes.
8. Remove and serve immediately.

Helpful Tips:

- Use the low-sodium tartar sauce recipe

found in Chapter 7 to go with this fish recipe.

- Other types of fish that can be used with this recipe include yellowtail, tilapia, and halibut.

Fish Stew

Total Prep & Cooking Time: 30 minutes

Makes: Three Helpings

Sodium: 73 mg

Protein: 28 gm

Fat: 9 gm

Sugar: 3 gm

Calories: 227

What you need:

- One tbsp. red pepper flakes
- Two cloves garlic, minced
- 4 oz. onion, chopped
- One lb. haddock fillets
- Two sticks celery, chopped
- One 4.5 oz. can tomatoes, diced, salt-free and undrained
- Two tbsp. olive oil

Steps:

1. Prepare the onion by removing the skin and chopping into small cubes. Scrub the celery and tomatoes and dice them together. Set to the side.
2. Use a hot skillet to warm the olive oil for about 30 seconds.
3. Blend the onion and garlic into the hot skillet for approximately 5 minutes.
4. Combine the tomatoes, red pepper flakes, and celery to the pan and adjust the heat down to slowly bubble for 10 more minutes.
5. Finally, for approximately ten minutes, heat the fish and remove from heat.

6. Serve immediately and enjoy!

Fried Rice

Total Prep & Cooking Time: 30 minutes

Makes: 4 Helpings

Sodium: 282 mg

Protein: 6 gm

Fat: 12 gm

Sugar: 4 gm

Calories: 225

What you need:

- One-half cup green bell pepper, chopped finely
- One-half cup scallion, chopped finely
- Two tbsp. soy sauce, low-sodium (See Helpful Tips)
- Three tbsp. olive oil
- Six oz. carrots, chopped finely
- One-half cup red bell pepper, chopped

finely
- Two-thirds cups brown rice, uncooked
- 4 oz. canned peas, drained
- Two large eggs
- One cup water
- One tbsp. sesame oil
- One-fourth cup parsley, chopped

Steps:

1. Heat a saucepan with the water and brown rice until it is bubbling.
2. Cover the saucepan and turn the burner off. Set to the side for 10 minutes.
3. In the meantime, thoroughly wash the bell peppers, carrots, and scallion.
4. Chop into very small sections and set to the side.
5. Heat a wok or skillet with the olive oil.
6. Distribute the brown rice into the skillet. Heat for about three minutes while tossing occasionally.

7. Combine the peas, bell peppers, carrots, and scallions into the skillet and fry for approximately 5 minutes, occasionally tossing.

8. Meanwhile, whip the eggs fully in a glass dish.

9. Create a hollow in the middle of the skillet and empty the egg into the indention and heat for about 60 seconds as the eggs start to set.

10. Blend the entire pan together and drizzle with sesame oil, soy sauce, and the chopped parsley.

11. Transfer to serving dishes and enjoy immediately!

Helpful Tip:

- In Chapter 7, there is a healthy low-sodium recipe for soy sauce.

Mexican Salad

Total Prep & Cooking Time: 25 minutes

Makes: One Salad

Sodium: 363 gm

Protein: 6 gm

Fat: 18 gm

Sugar: 5 gm

Calories: 283

What you need:

- One-half cup lettuce, chopped
- Eight oz. tomatoes
- One scallion, chopped
- Three tbsp. olive oil
- One oz. ground beef, lean
- One/eight package of taco seasoning (See Helpful Tips below)
- Three-fourths cup water

- One oz. cheddar cheese, sharp

Steps:

1. Brown the meat in a skillet with the warmed olive oil for approximately 8 minutes until fully cooked. Break the meat into small chunks with a wooden spatula.
2. In the meantime, scrub the scallion thoroughly and chop along with the lettuce. Set to the side.
3. Remove the pan from the burner and strain the liquid out of the pan.
4. Return to the burner and blend the water and taco seasoning until combined.
5. Let the mixture reduce for about 10 minutes.
6. Meanwhile, wash the tomatoes and scallions thoroughly. Cut into large chunks along with the lettuce. Transfer to a serving dish.
7. Distribute the cooked meat after it has properly reduced and top with the shredded cheddar cheese.
8. Serve while hot and enjoy!

Helpful Tips:

- There is a healthy recipe alternative for taco seasoning in Chapter 7.

- The French dressing recipe found also in Chapter 7 goes well with this dish.

- To add more variety, you can add one/eight cup of corn or black beans to this recipe.

Minestrone Soup

Total Prep & Cooking Time: 30 minutes

Makes: 4 Helpings

Sodium: 125 gm

Protein: 27gm

Fat: 8gm

Sugar: 17 gm

Calories: 490

What you need:

- Four cups chicken broth, low-salt (See Helpful Tip below)
- One-half cup onion, chopped
- Three tsp. olive oil
- One carrot, diced
- Two celery stalks, chopped
- Sixteen oz. can garbanzo beans, low-sodium, drained and washed

- One small zucchini
- One-half cup spinach, chopped
- Four oz. whole wheat pasta shells
- One clove garlic, minced
- Two tbsp. basil, chopped

Steps:

1. Wash the vegetables thoroughly and chop into small sections, keeping them separate. Set to the side.
2. Warm a skillet with the olive oil for approximately half a minute.
3. Empty the carrots, celery and onion into the hot skillet and brown for approximately 5 minutes.
4. Combine the minced garlic to the skillet and incorporate well.
5. Blend the tomatoes, garbanzo beans, chicken broth, and pasta into the skillet and heat until boiling.
6. Bring down the heat for the dish to reduce for about 10 minutes.
7. Lastly, combine the zucchini into the pan

and use a lid to cover for an additional 5 minutes.

8. Enjoy immediately.

Helpful Tip:

- Included in Chapter 7 is a homemade recipe for low-sodium chicken broth.

Mushroom Fajitas

Total Prep & Cooking Time: 25 minutes

Makes: 3 Helpings

Sodium: 193 mg

Protein: 4 gm

Fat: 1 gm

Sugar: 10 gm

Calories: 102

What you need:

- One tbsp. olive oil
- Two Portobello mushrooms
- One tbsp. lime juice
- Three-fourths cup onion, sliced
- One tsp. cumin seasoning
- Three bell peppers, your choice of color and sliced
- One-fourth tsp. salt

- Three-fourths tsp. garlic powder
- One tsp. smoked paprika seasoning

Steps:

1. Scrub the mushrooms and bell peppers well. Slice the bell peppers into long strips.

2. Remove the skin from the onion and chop into slices as well.

3. Warm the oil in a hot frying pan and combine the mushrooms, onions, and bell peppers.

4. Season with the smoked paprika, salt, cumin, and garlic powder while frying for approximately 15 minutes. Toss occasionally.

5. In the meantime, crush the avocado in a container and blend the juice of the lime and set to the side.

6. Transfer the content of the skillet to a serving plate and top with the crushed avocado and enjoy while hot.

Helpful Tip:

- If you would like to add more protein, you can fry 16 oz. of low-sodium black beans in the skillet during the last 5 minutes of frying.

Orange Chicken

Total Prep & Cooking Time: 30 minutes

Makes: Two Helpings

Sodium: 40Two mg

Protein: 34 gm

Fat: 8 gm

Sugar: 12 gm

Calories: 400

What you need:

- Three-fourths cup natural orange juice

- One cup water
- Two cloves garlic, peeled
- One tbsp. soy sauce, low-sodium (See Helpful Tip below)
- Two tsp. ginger, grated
- Eight oz. chicken breast, no bones or skin
- Two tsp. red pepper flakes
- One tsp. sesame oil
- Six oz. carrots, sliced thinly
- Three tsp. orange zest
- Two tsp. cornstarch
- Two scallions, sliced
- One-third cup brown rice, uncooked
- One tsp. red pepper flakes

Steps:

1. Warm a saucepan with the brown rice and water until it is bubbling.
2. Cover the pan and turn the burner off. Set to the side for 10 minutes.
3. In the meantime, blend the orange juice, garlic, soy sauce, ginger, cornstarch, and the orange zest until combined. Set aside.

4. Chop the chicken into small cubes.
5. Remove the skin from the onions and slice into thin sections. Thoroughly wash the carrot and cut into small slices. Set to the side.
6. Use a skillet to heat the sesame oil for about 20 seconds. Combine the chicken and toss occasionally for approximately 7 minutes until brown.
7. Empty the carrots into the skillet and heat for another 5 minutes while occasionally tossing.
8. Transfer the mixed sauce to the hot pan and reduce for approximately 5 minutes.
9. Spoon the brown rice into serving bowls and finish the dish with the chicken on top.
10. Sprinkle the sliced onions and red pepper flakes over the meal.
11. Serve immediately and enjoy!

Helpful Tip:

- In Chapter 7, you will discover the low-sodium recipe for soy sauce.

Veggie Jambalaya

Total Prep & Cooking Time: 30 minutes

Makes: 4 Helpings

Sodium: 58 mg

Protein: 3 gm

Fat: 6 gm

Sugar: 4 gm

Calories: 158

What you need:

- One-fourth tsp. salt
- Two cloves garlic, chopped finely
- One-eight tsp. cayenne pepper
- One bay leaf
- Two-thirds medium onion, chopped
- One small jalapeno, chopped finely
- One-third tsp. thyme seasoning
- Two medium stalks celery, chopped

- One large tomato, chopped
- Two-thirds tsp. paprika seasoning
- Four tsp. olive oil
- One-third tsp. oregano seasoning
- Two cups vegetable broth, low-salt (See Helpful Tips below)
- Two-thirds tsp. garlic powder
- One-half cup brown rice, long-grain and uncooked
- Two-thirds tsp. Worcestershire sauce (See Helpful Tips below)
- One-fourth tsp. black pepper
- Two-thirds medium green bell pepper

Steps:

1. Thoroughly scrub the bell pepper, celery, and tomato. Slice the top of the bell pepper off and cut in half. Remove the seeds and discard.
2. Take the outer skin off of the onion.
3. Chop the bell pepper, celery, tomato, jalapeno, and onion into small sections and set

to the side divided.

4. Heat a deep pot with the olive oil and warm the celery, onion, and bell pepper for approximately 5 minutes.

5. Blend the Worcestershire sauce, pepper, oregano, thyme, cayenne, garlic powder, salt, bay leaf, tomatoes, chili, and garlic into the pot. Heat for about 60 seconds.

6. Then, combine the vegetable broth and rice into the stew and turn the burner down.

7. Reduce for approximately 23 minutes and remove from the heat.

8. Spoon into individual serving dishes and enjoy while hot.

Helpful Tips:

- Look in Chapter 7 to find the alternative healthy low-sodium recipes for Worcestershire sauce and the vegetable broth.

- Alternatively, you can substitute soy sauce for the Worcestershire sauce.

- Any leftovers can be placed in a lidded tub in the fridge for 4 days.

Oven Baked Sea Bass

Total Prep & Cooking Time: 15 minutes

Makes: 4 Helpings

Sodium: 395 mg

Protein: 40 gm

Fat: 11 gm

Sugar: 0 gm

Calories: 271

What you need:

- One-fourth tsp. salt
- Four 6 oz. sea bass fillets, descaled and deboned
- Two tbsp. olive oil
- One-fourth tsp. black pepper

Steps:

1. Adjust the temperature of the stove to 400° Fahrenheit. Layer a flat sheet with foil and set the fish onto the tray.

2. Remove any extra moisture from the fish and coat with the oil fully with a brush.

3. Dust with the pepper and salt on both sides.

4. Heat in the stove for approximately 10 minutes and serve immediately.

Helpful Tip:

- You can use the healthy Thai Marinade recipe in Chapter 7 with this fish recipe. Make sure you cut the fish along the meat and place in a lidded container with the marinade for approximately three hours in the refrigerator before following the cooking methods above.

Quinoa Salad

Total Prep & Cooking Time: 5 minutes

Makes: One Salad

Sodium: 142 mg

Protein: 9 gm

Fat: 7 gm

Sugar: 1 gm

Calories: 268

What you need:

- One oz. corn
- Two oz. onion, chopped
- One-half tbsp. lime juice, separated
- 4 oz. water
- One-half tsp. olive oil
- Two oz. quinoa, uncooked
- One oz. sour cream, fat-free
- Two-thirds cup shredded lettuce

- One-fourth red bell pepper, diced
- One oz. canned black beans, low-sodium, rinsed and drained
- One-fourth clove garlic, minced

Steps:

1. Wash the bell pepper thoroughly and dice into small sections. Set to the side.
2. Use a saucepan to warm the 4 ounces of water under bubbling.
3. Empty the quinoa into a strainer with mesh and wash thoroughly under the tap with cold water.
4. Transfer the quinoa to the hot saucepan and adjust the heat down to slowly bubble for approximately 10 minutes.
5. Blend in one-fourth tablespoon of the lime juice and place a lid on top of the saucepan.
6. Empty the last one-fourth tablespoon of lime juice and the sour cream in a separate dish and set to the side.
7. Use a non-stick pan to warm the olive oil. Combine the bell pepper and onions to the hot

oil and heat for approximately 5 minutes while occasionally stirring.

8. The blend the minced garlic into the pan and heat for another 60 seconds.

9. Finally, combine the corn and the black beans to the skillet and heat for an additional 4 minutes.

10. Empty the lettuce into a dish and distribute the sour cream and black bean mixture over the top.

11. Toss to completely integrate and serve immediately.

Helpful Tip:

- Try the low-sodium healthy dressing recipes found in Chapter 7 to top your salad with Yogurt, Italian, French, Ranch, Thousand Island, or Avocado Dressing.

Sloppy Joe Sandwich

Total Prep & Cooking Time: 30 minutes

Makes: 4 Burgers

Sodium: 467 mg

Protein: 30 gm

Fat: 8 gm

Sugar: 8 gm

Calories: 333

What you need:

- One-fourth tsp. salt
- 12 oz. chicken, ground
- Two-thirds tbsp. brown sugar
- Two oz. red onion, diced
- One-third tsp. garlic powder
- One-half cup ketchup, low-sodium (See Helpful Tip below)
- Two oz. red pepper, diced

- Four whole wheat hamburger buns
- One tsp. mustard (See Helpful Tip below)
- Two oz. yellow pepper, diced
- One-fourth tsp. black pepper
- Three tbsp. olive oil

Steps:

1. Wash and slice the onion and bell peppers into tiny cubes.

2. Warm the oil in a frying pan for about half a minute before combining the chopped vegetables and ground chicken for approximately 8 minutes.

3. Remove the extra fluid in the pan and put back onto the burner.

4. Adjust the temperature to simmer and blend in the garlic powder, brown sugar, mustard, and ketchup until fully incorporated.

5. Leave to heat from an additional two minutes and spice with pepper and salt.

6. Evenly spoon the mixture onto the hamburger buns and serve while hot!

Helpful Tip:

- You will find a healthy alternative recipe to make homemade low-sodium ketchup and mustard in Chapter 7.

Spaghetti with Vegetables

Total Prep & Cooking Time: 30 minutes

Makes: 4 Helpings

Sodium: 395 mg

Protein: 7 gm

Fat: 5 gm

Sugar: 4 gm

Calories: 185

What you need:

- One-fourth tsp. black
- Two cloves garlic, minced
- Three cups spinach
- pepper
- One-fourth tsp. red pepper flakes
- 8 oz. button mushrooms, sliced
- One-fourth tsp. salt
- Two cups vegetable broth, low-salt (See

Helpful Tip below)

- One4.5 oz. can tomatoes, salt-free and diced
- One0 oz. spaghetti noodles, whole wheat
- One-half cup yellow onion, chopped
- Two tsp. olive oil
- One-half cup Parmesan cheese

Steps:

1. Take the outer skin off of the onion and chop roughly.
2. Remove the excess dirt from the mushrooms and slice.
3. In a deep stockpot, combine the olive oil, mushrooms, and onion and warm for approximately 6 minutes.
4. Season with the salt, garlic, red pepper flakes, and pepper for another half minute.
5. Raise the heat on the burner and blend the vegetable broth and tomatoes until boiling.
6. Turn down the burner to low and empty the noodles into the pot. Use a lid to cover for approximately 5 minutes while simmering.

7. Combine the spinach and heat for another 60 seconds while stirring to integrate.

8. Turn the burner completely off and wait for about three minutes for the mixture to complete the baking process.

9. Blend the parmesan cheese into the spaghetti and serve while still hot.

Helpful Tip:

- You will find a healthy low-sodium vegetable broth recipe in Chapter 7.

Tuna Salad

Total Prep & Cooking Time: 10 minutes

Makes: 4 Helpings

Sodium: 399 mg

Protein: 18 gm

Fat: 4 gm

Sugar: 1 gm

Calories: 128

What you need:

- One-fourth tsp. garlic powder
- One-half avocado, diced
- 12 oz. canned tuna, in water and drained
- One-fourth tsp. salt
- Two tbsp. red onion, minced
- One tsp. lemon juice
- One-third cup Greek yogurt
- Two tsp. mustard, low-sodium (See

Helpful Tips below)
- One stalk celery, minced
- One-fourth tsp. black pepper

Steps:

1. Thoroughly wash the celery. Slice into very small sections.

2. Prepare the onion by removing the skin and chop into small chunks.

3. Slice the avocado in half and slice one half into cubes.

4. Fully drain the tuna to remove as much moisture as possible.

5. In a glass dish, blend the red onion, celery, and tuna until incorporated.

6. Combine the mustard, lemon juice, avocado, and Greek yogurt until blended.

7. Spice with the pepper, garlic powder, and salt.

8. Spoon into a serving dish or serve with toasted whole wheat bread. Enjoy immediately.

Helpful Tips:

- See Chapter 7 for a recipe for low-sodium mustard that can be used in this recipe.

- Store this salad in the fridge for approximately 5 days in a lidded tub.

Turkey Panini

Total Prep & Cooking Time: 20 minutes

Makes: 4 Sandwiches

Sodium: 519 mg

Protein: 14 gm

Fat: 13 gm

Sugar: 2 gm

Calories: 229

What you need:

- Two tbsp. olive oil
- Eight slices whole wheat bread
- Two tbsp. vinegar, balsamic
- One clove garlic
- Four slices mozzarella cheese
- Three cups baby spinach
- Four slices turkey breast, deli
- One-half cup onion, red

Steps:

1. Prepare the garlic and red onion by removing the skins. Mince the garlic and section the onion into slices.

2. Blend the balsamic vinegar, olive oil, and garlic in a glass dish.

3. Use a pastry brush to apply the mixture on each slice of bread on only one side.

4. Arrange one piece of bread with the oil side directly on the electric sandwich grill and layer the spinach, onion, slice of mozzarella, and turkey.

5. Finish with another slice of bread with the

oil side on the top of the sandwich.

    6. Press the sandwich together by closing the grill and heat for approximately three minutes until the cheese melts.

    7. Repeat steps 4 through 6 for the remaining sandwiches.

    8. Serve while still warm and enjoy!

Turkey Tacos

Total Prep & Cooking Time: 20 minutes

Makes: 4 Tacos

Sodium: 305 mg

Protein: 18gm

Fat: 13 gm

Sugar: 1 gm

Calories: 242

What you need:

- One clove garlic, minced
- One-fourth tsp. salt
- One-third tsp. brown sugar
- Four whole grain taco shells
- One-third tsp. olive oil
- One-third cup onion, chopped finely
- One-fourth cup chicken broth, low-salt(See Helpful Tips below)
- One-fourth tsp. black pepper
- Two oz. cilantro, chopped
- Three-fourths tbsp. chili powder, salt-free
- 8 oz. turkey, ground
- Three-fourths tsp. cider vinegar
- One-third tsp. oregano seasoning
- Two oz. tomato sauce, low-sodium (See Helpful Tips below)
- One-third tsp. ground cumin

Steps:

1. Remove the outer layer of the onion and discard. Chop the onion into small chunks.

2. Dissolve the olive oil in a hot frying pan and brown the onion in the oil for approximately

5 minutes.

3. Combine the oregano, cumin, garlic, and chili powder to the pan and heat for half a minute.

4. Blend the ground turkey into the skillet and heat for another 4 minutes. Use a wooden spatula to crumble the meat and combine thoroughly.

5. Finally, mix the tomato sauce, vinegar, and brown sugar in the skillet and allow to reduce for approximately four minutes.

6. Adjust the burner to turn it off. Blend the pepper, cilantro, and salt in the pan.

7. Put the mixture in the taco shells and complete with your favorite toppings. Serve and enjoy!

Helpful Tips:

- Included in Chapter 7 is a homemade recipe for low-sodium chicken broth and the marinara sauce.

- Avoid using ground turkey that is virtually fat-free as the taco filling will end up too dry otherwise.

- Healthy ideas for toppings include Greek yogurt, avocado, tomatoes, and cheddar cheese.

Vegetable Soup

Total Prep & Cooking Time: 30 minutes

Makes: 4 Helpings

Sodium: 513 mg

Protein: 12 gm

Fat: 2 gm

Sugar: 2 gm

Calories: 275

What you need:

- One bay leaf
- Three medium russet potatoes
- One-half cup water
- Four medium carrots, chopped
- One tsp. oregano seasoning
- Two-thirds cup yellow onion, chopped
- One tsp. parsley seasoning
- Seventeen oz. canned diced tomatoes,

salt-free and undrained
- Two medium celery stalks, chopped
- One and one-third cups yellow corn, frozen
- Twenty-one oz. vegetable broth, low-salt (See Helpful Tip below)
- One and one-third cups green peas, frozen

Steps:

1. Thoroughly clean the carrots, celery, and potatoes. Chop the carrots and celery into small sections and set to the side.

2. Utilize a peeler or knife to take off the skin of the potatoes. Chop into cubes and set aside.

3. In a deep pot, integrate the celery, carrots, onion, and the water and heat for approximately 6 minutes while occasionally tossing.

4. Blend the parsley, oregano, and bay leaf into the pot and incorporate fully.

5. Empty the diced tomatoes and juice, corn, peas, chopped potatoes, and the vegetable

broth.

6. If there is not enough water to cover the vegetables, add until they are covered by half an inch.

7. Warm and when the stew starts to bubble, adjust the temperature of the burner to low.

8. Lightly bubble for about 35 minutes while occasionally stirring.

9. Turn the burner completely off and take the bay leaf out of the pot.

10. Spoon into individual serving dishes and enjoy while hot.

Helpful Tip:

- Use the recipe for the low-sodium vegetable broth located in Chapter 7.

Zucchini Frittata

Total Prep& Cooking Time: 20 minutes

Makes: 4 Servings

Sodium: 346 mg

Protein: 11 gm

Fat: 13 gm

Sugar: 2 gm

Calories: 182

What you need:

- 6 large eggs
- 8 oz. zucchini
- One-half onion, sliced
- One and one-half tbsp. olive oil
- 4 oz. sweet corn, drained
- One-half tsp. salt

Steps:

1. Preheat your stove to heat at 400° Fahrenheit.
2. Take the outer layer off of the onion and slice thinly.
3. Warm a heavy duty frying pan with the oil and combine the onions in the pan. Caramelize for approximately 5 minutes.
4. Use a glass dish to whip the salt and the egg until integrated fully.
5. Combine the sweet corn and the zucchini into the skillet and toss for about half a minute. Then empty the eggs into the pan.
6. Move the pan to the hot stove and warm for 10 minutes.
7. Then adjust the stove to broil and leave the pan for an additional minute.
8. Remove the cast iron pan and cut into 4 sections.
9. Transfer to serving plates and enjoy while hot.

Chapter 6: Dinner Recipes

Baked Salmon

Total Prep & Cooking Time: 40 minutes

Makes: 4 Helpings

Sodium: 270 mg

Protein: 27 gm

Fat: 14 gm

Sugar: 0 gm

Calories: 264

What you need:

- Two-thirds tbsp. maple syrup
- One-fourth tsp. black pepper
- One and one-third tbsp. soy sauce, low-sodium (See Helpful Tip below)
- olive oil cooking spray
- One-fourth tsp. salt

- Twenty oz. salmon fillet
- Two-thirds tbsp. honey

Steps:

1. Prepare a glass baking dish by coating with olive oil spray.
2. Transfer the salmon to the baking dish and ensure that all moisture is removed.
3. Use a brush to transfer the soy sauce to the entire fillet and dust with the pepper and salt.
4. Marinate on the counter for approximately 15 minutes.
5. Adjust the stove temperature to heat at 425° Fahrenheit. Heat the fish for 7 minutes.
6. In the meantime, blend the maple syrup and honey in a glass dish.
7. Apply the honey mixture on the fish with the pastry brush.
8. Heat for an additional 8 minutes and remove from the stove.

9. Transfer to a serving platter and enjoy immediately.

Helpful Tip:

- Look in Chapter 7 for a healthy low-sodium recipe for the soy sauce and, if you prefer, tartar sauce.

Beef Stroganoff

Total Prep & Cooking Time: 45 minutes

Makes: 4 Helpings

Sodium: 458 mg

Protein: 42 gm

Fat: 11 gm

Sugar: 4 gm

Calories: 442

What you need:

- One cup sour cream, fat-free
- Four cloves garlic, crushed
- Sixteen oz. fettuccine noodles, whole wheat
- One lb. mushrooms, sliced
- Four tbsp. margarine, separated
- One cup onion, chopped
- Two tbsp. whole wheat flour
- One and one-half lb. beef fillet steaks, lean
- Two tsp. mustard, low-sodium (See Helpful Tips below)
- One-half tsp. salt, separated
- Two cups vegetable broth, low-salt (See Helpful Tips below)
- One tsp. paprika seasoning
- Three tsp. Worcestershire sauce, low-sodium (See Helpful Tips below)
- One-half tsp. black pepper, separated
- Sixteen cups water
- One-third cup white wine, dry

Steps:

1. Prepare the onion by removing the skin and dicing into small sections. Set aside.

2. Rub any extra dirt off of the mushrooms and slice. Set to the side.

3. Warm a deep pot with the water and the whole wheat fettuccine noodles with one-fourth teaspoon of the salt for approximately 10 minutes.

4. In the meantime, chop the beef into small cubes and dust with one-fourth teaspoon of pepper.

5. Liquefy two tablespoons of the margarine in a big skillet and transfer the cubed meat into the pan. Fry the meat for approximately 8 minutes while tossing occasionally to fully brown.

6. Remove the water from the cooked pasta and set to the side.

7. Use a spoon with holes to distribute the cooked meat to a platter and keep to the side.

8. Dissolve the leftover two tablespoons of margarine in the hot frying pan and fry the onions for approximately 5 minutes to caramelize.

9. Blend the garlic into the pan and heat for

an additional half minute.

10. Then combine the mushrooms with the onions and fry for about 4 minutes.

11. Season the vegetables with the paprika and mustard and empty the wine into the skillet and heat for another 6 minutes, occasionally tossing and rubbing the base of the pan with a spatula that is wooden.

12. Meanwhile, blend the Worcestershire sauce, flour, and vegetable broth in a glass dish until there are no lumps present.

13. Empty the sauce into the skillet and bring to a slow bubble for approximately 5 minutes while occasionally stirring.

14. Transfer the cooked meat to the skillet and spice with the remaining one-fourth teaspoons of the pepper and salt.

15. Turn the burner down to the setting of low and blend the sour cream into the skillet. Heat for an additional two minutes.

16. Distribute the cooked noodles into the pan and cover fully with the sauce.

17. Spoon into serving dishes and enjoy immediately.

Helpful Tips:

- Look in Chapter 7 for the recipe for a low-sodium Worcestershire sauce, mustard, and chicken broth.

- You can substitute several varieties of beef for the fillet steaks including flank steak, tenderloin, or sirloin.

Black Bean Burgers

Total Prep & Cooking Time: 45 minutes

Makes: 4 Burgers

Sodium: 458 mg

Protein: 12 gm

Fat: 1 gm

Sugar: 1 gm

Calories: 213

What you need:

- Twenty-four oz. black beans, low-sodium, drained and washed
- Three-fourths tsp. maple syrup
- One tsp. paprika seasoning
- Three-fourths tbsp. hot sauce
- One two-thirds tsp. garlic, chopped finely
- Two-thirds cup panko breadcrumbs
- One two-thirds tbsp. soy sauce, low-

sodium (See Helpful Tips below)
- Three tsp. olive oil

Steps:

1. Combine the black beans, maple syrup, paprika, hot sauce, garlic, breadcrumbs, and soy sauce in a glass dish.

2. Mix until incorporated by hand and refrigerate for approximately 5 minutes.

3. Warm the oil in a frying pan.

4. Remove from the fridge and form 4 individual patties by hand.

5. Arrange the burgers to the hot skillet and heat for about 10 minutes before flipping to the other side.

6. Warm for an additional 10 minutes and serve as is or on a whole wheat burger bun. Enjoy!

Helpful Tips:

- Find the low-sodium healthy recipe alternative to soy sauce in Chapter 7.

- You can also cook these on the grill.

- Varieties that you add use to spice up this recipe is to combine a one-half cup of onions or corn.

Chicken Kabobs

Total Prep & Cooking Time: 45 minutes

Makes: 2 Helpings

Sodium: 72 mg

Protein: 27 gm

Fat: 10 gm

Sugar: 3 gm

Calories: 228

What you need:

- One-fourth cup parsley seasoning
- olive oil cooking spray
- One cup cherry tomatoes
- 8 oz. chicken breast, no bones or skins
- One tbsp. lime juice
- Three tsp. vinegar, red wine
- One-fourth cup cilantro seasoning
- One-half tsp. black pepper

- One tbsp. water
- Two cloves garlic
- Three tsp. olive oil
- Three tsp. oregano seasoning
- One-half tsp. red pepper flakes, crushed

Steps:

1. Use a food blender to pulse the cilantro, oregano, red pepper flakes, garlic, pepper, olive oil, and water for about half a minute.
2. Then combine the vinegar, lime juice, and parsley to the blender and pulse for another half minute.
3. Divide the chicken into tiny cubes and transfer to a large ziplock bag.
4. Divide the sauce into half and ladle into the ziplock bag and agitate to fully cover the cubed chicken. Refrigerate for approximately 25 minutes.
5. Place the leftover sauce in a lidded tube and transfer to the fridge until dinner time.
6. Heat the grill to prepare for cooking at the medium setting.

7. After the half-hour has elapsed, carefully take the chicken out of the bag and toss out the sauce.

8. Layer the tomatoes and chicken onto the skewers until full.

9. Apply a coat of olive oil spray to the spears and move to the grill.

10. Heat for approximately three minutes before turning over for another two minutes.

11. Lower the heat and continue to grill for approximately 12 minutes and remove to a serving plate.

12. Immediately serve with the sauce and enjoy!

Helpful Tips:

- If you have the wooden variety of spears, immerse them in tepid water for approximately 10 minutes prior to using.

- You may use any vinegar in this recipe in

place of the red wine vinegar or substitute lime juice instead.

- To add variety to this recipe, consider layering mushrooms or zucchini to the skewers.

Crunchy Fried Chicken

Total Prep & Cooking Time: 45 minutes

Makes: 4 Helpings

Sodium: 481 mg

Protein: 45 gm

Fat: 7 gm

Sugar: 1 gm

Calories: 540

What you need:

- One-fourth tsp. salt
- One/eight tsp. dry mustard seasoning
- One-half tsp. cayenne pepper
- Two oz. cornmeal
- One-half tsp. paprika seasoning
- Two oz. cornflakes, crumbled
- Four chicken breasts, boneless and skinless

- Two tbsp. whole wheat flour
- olive oil cooking spray
- Two oz. buttermilk, low-fat
- One tsp. garlic powder

Steps:

1. Set the stove to heat at 375° Fahrenheit. Apply a coat of olive oil spray over a 9-inch glass baking dish.
2. Empty the buttermilk into a glass dish.
3. In an additional dish, blend the cornflakes, cornmeal, and flour with a whisk to integrate.
4. Season with the mustard, cayenne pepper, paprika, garlic powder, and salt and combine fully.
5. Immerse one chicken breast first in the buttermilk and then into the cornflakes to completely cover the meat. Make sure the chicken is not dripping by removing any excess batter.
6. Transfer the coated chicken to the prepped baking dish.
7. Repeat steps 5 and 6 for the remaining

chicken.

8. Apply the olive oil spray to the chicken and heat in the stove for half an hour.

9. Remove and enjoy immediately while hot.

Herbed Oven Roasted Veggies

Total Prep & Cooking Time: 60 minutes

Makes: 4 Helpings

Sodium: 29 mg

Protein: 3 gm

Fat: 6 gm

Sugar: 0 gm

Calories: 135

What you need:

- One-half large Vidalia onion
- 4 cloves garlic
- One medium beet

- olive oil cooking spray
- One-half pound Russet potatoes
- Two medium carrots
- One-fourth tsp. black pepper, separated
- Two medium zucchini
- One-half red bell pepper
- Three tsp. rosemary, chopped and separated
- Two sprigs rosemary
- One and one-half tbsp. olive oil, separated

Steps:

1. Scrub the potatoes, carrots, zucchini, beet, and bell pepper. Remove the skin of the onion, carrots, and beet. Remove the seeds from the bell pepper.

2. Chop the beet, onion, zucchini, carrots, and potatoes into large cubes and set to the side.

3. Set the stove temperature to heat at 400° Fahrenheit and move the racks to the lowest

setting. Apply the olive oil spray to two separate flat sheets with a rim and set to the side.

4. Blend the onion, garlic, zucchini, carrots, peppers, potatoes, and one tablespoon of the olive oil until fully coated.

5. Season with one/eight teaspoon of rosemary and one-half teaspoon of the black pepper that is chopped and blend well.

6. Use an additional dish to combine the beets, the leftover olive oil, the last one/eight teaspoon of pepper and the leftover a one-half teaspoon of chopped rosemary. Coat the beets evenly by tossing.

7. Evenly distribute the prepared vegetables between the two prepped flat sheets and heat for 20 minutes.

8. Flip the vegetables over and continue to heat for an additional 22 minutes.

9. Take the dish out from the stove, garnish with the rosemary sprigs and serve immediately.

Lintel Stew

Total Prep & Cooking Time: 45 minutes

Makes: 4 Helpings

Sodium: 231 mg

Protein: 16 gm

Fat: 1 gm

Sugar: 10 gm

Calories: 248

What you need:

- Three carrots, peeled and chopped
- Two cloves garlic, minced
- Three-fourths cup yellow bell pepper, chopped
- One cup dried red lentils, rinsed
- 5 cups vegetable broth, low-salt (see

Helpful Tip below)
- One cup yellow onion, chopped
- One4 oz. can tomatoes, low-sodium and diced
- olive oil cooking spray
- One-half cup celery, chopped

Steps:

1. Thoroughly scrub the bell pepper, celery, and carrots. Chop them roughly and set to the side.
2. Cover a deep pot with olive oil spray and warm on the burner.
3. Caramelize the garlic and onions for approximately three minutes.
4. Combine the lentils, vegetable broth, and tomatoes and heat to make the water bubble.
5. Adjust the temperature down to allow the pot to slowly bubble and put a lid on the top.
6. Continue to heat for approximately half an hour.

7. Serve will still hot and enjoy!

Helpful Tip:

- Included in Chapter 7 is a homemade recipe for low-sodium vegetable broth.

Mashed Potatoes

Total Prep & Cooking Time: 40 minutes

Makes: 4 Helpings

Sodium: 81 mg

Protein: 6 gm

Fat: 7 gm

Sugar: 0 gm

Calories: 184

What you need:

- One-third cup sour cream, low-fat
- Three and one-fourth garlic cloves, halved
- One-third cup vegetable broth, low-salt (See Helpful Tip below)
- One-fourth tsp. black pepper
- One and two-thirds lb. russet potatoes
- cold water
- One and two-thirds tbsp. margarine
- One-half tsp. salt, separated

Steps:

1. Scrub and thoroughly clean the potatoes. Use a vegetable peeler to remove the skins and then chop into large cubes.

2. In the meantime, fill a deep pot a little more than halfway with water and one-fourth teaspoon of the salt.

3. When the water starts to bubble, transfer the cubed potatoes into the pot along with the garlic. Use a top to cover and heat for approximately 15 minutes.

4. Remove the water from the pot ensuring the garlic and potatoes remain and put the top back on. Let it rest for about 10 minutes.

5. Crush the potatoes with a masher and blend the margarine, broth, and sour cream into the pot.

6. Spice with the pepper and the leftover one-fourth teaspoon of salt and serve while still hot.

Helpful Tip:

- Find the healthy alternative recipe for low-sodium vegetable broth in Chapter 7.

Pumpkin Soup

Total Prep & Cooking Time: 35 minutes

Makes: 4 Helpings

Sodium: 530 gm

Protein: 5 gm

Fat: 2 gm

Sugar: 6 gm

Calories: 128

What you need:

- One-third cup sour cream, fat-free
- One-fourth tsp. black pepper
- One chicken bouillon cube, crushed
- Three-fourths cup onion, chopped
- Two and one-half cloves garlic, crushed
- Twenty oz. pumpkin meat, seeds removed and cubed

- One-fourth tsp. salt
- Two and one-half cups vegetable broth, low-salt (See Helpful Tips below)
- One oz. carrot, peeled and diced
- Eight oz. potato, peeled and diced

Steps:

1. Prepare the pumpkin by removing the seeds and slicing the meat into cubes.
2. Thoroughly scrub the potato and carrot and use a vegetable peeler to remove the skin. Chop them into small sections and set to the side.
3. Remove the skin of the onion and discard. Roughly chop the onion into small cubes and set aside.
4. Combine the pumpkin meat, onion, carrot, potato, and vegetable broth in a deep pot.
5. Blend the chicken bouillon cube, salt, crushed garlic, and pepper into the pot and integrate completely.
6. Heat for approximately 15 minutes until you can slice the vegetables with a fork.

7. Remove from the burner and use an electrical blender until fully cream.

8. Finally, blend the sour cream into the mixture and serve while hot.

Helpful Tips:

- Find the recipe for the healthy low-sodium version of vegetable broth in Chapter 7.

- If you would like to spruce the soup up, you can garnish with one-third cup of bacon bits or chopped parsley.

Red Beans & Rice

Total Prep & Cooking Time: 45 minutes

Makes: 4 Helpings

Sodium: 254 mg

Protein: 13 gm

Fat: 1 gm

Sugar: 6 gm

Calories: 329

What you need:

- 8 oz. tomato sauce, salt-free (See Helpful Tip below)
- One and one-half cups brown rice, uncooked
- olive oil cooking spray
- 32 oz. can dark red kidney beans, low-salt and undrained
- One cup frozen mixed vegetables, chopped

- One-fourth tsp. garlic powder
- One-half tsp. Italian seasoning
- One-half cup water
- Three tsp. Cajun seasoning
- One 4.5 oz. diced tomatoes, salt-free and undrained

Steps:

1. Coat a frying pan with the oil spray and sauté the mixed vegetables for about Three minutes.
2. Fully blend the kidney beans with the juice, tomatoes with the juice, water, garlic powder, Italian seasoning, tomato sauce, brown rice, and Cajun seasoning into the pan.
3. When the mixture starts to bubble, turn the burner to the setting of low.
4. Use a lid and reduce for approximately 15 minutes and remove from heat.
5. Wait about 5 minutes before serving and enjoy!

Helpful Tip:

- You can use the healthy low-sodium marinara sauce recipe in place of the tomato paste. It is found in Chapter 7.

Sesame Chicken

Total Prep & Cooking Time: 35 minutes

Makes: 4 Helpings

Sodium: 527 mg

Protein: 28 gm

Fat: 6 gm

Sugar: 3 gm

Calories: 226

What you need:

- One tbsp. water
- One-fourth tsp. black pepper
- Two tbsp. sesame seeds
- One lb. chicken breast, no bones or skin
- Three tsp. maple syrup
- One tsp. ginger root, minced
- Three tsp. dry sherry
- One-fourth tsp. salt

- Two tbsp. whole wheat flour
- Three tsp. soy sauce, low-sodium (See Helpful Tip below)
- Two tsp. olive oil

Steps:

1. Empty the sesame seeds in a hot frying pan and heat for about two minutes when they start to pop. Remove to a glass dish and set to the side.
2. In another glass dish, blend the ginger, sherry, maple syrup, water, and soy sauce until integrated. Set aside.
3. Slice the chicken into small strips and heat the olive oil in the same skillet.
4. Use a third dish to combine the pepper, flour, chicken, and salt making sure the meat is completely covered.
5. Remove any extra flour from the chicken and transfer to the hot oil.
6. Fry for approximately three minutes before turning over. Continue to heat for another two minutes.

7. Blend the sauce previously combined to the skillet and allow to come to a slow bubble for approximately three minutes to reduce.

8. Remove the chicken to individual plates and coat with the toasted sesame seeds.

9. Serve immediately and enjoy!

Helpful Tip:

- Find the healthy low-sodium soy sauce recipe in Chapter 7.

Thai Vegetable Curry

Total Prep & Cooking Time: 45 minutes

Makes: 4 Helpings

Sodium: 473 mg

Protein: 8 gm

Fat: 11 gm

Sugar: 9 gm

Calories: 340

What you need:

- Two tsp. lime juice
- One cup white onion, chopped
- Two and one-half cups water, separated
- Ten oz. brown rice, long-grain and uncooked
- One-fourth tsp. salt

- Three tsp. olive oil
- One tbsp. soy sauce, low-sodium (See Helpful Tips below)
- Three tsp. ginger, finely grated
- Fourteen oz. canned light coconut milk
- One cup carrot
- Two tbsp. Thai curry paste, red
- One and one-half tsp. brown sugar
- Two bell peppers, your choice of color and sliced
- One and one-half cups kale
- Two cloves garlic, crushed

Steps:

1. Scrub the carrot and bell peppers well. Peel and chop the carrot into thin diagonal

slices. Slice the bell peppers into strips and set to the side.

2. Prepare the kale by discarding the hard ribs and then chopping finely. Set aside.

3. Remove the skin of the onion and roughly chop. Set to the side.

4. Warm a saucepan with two cups of the water and brown rice until the water is bubbling.

5. Cover the saucepan and turn the heat off. Allow to reduce for ten minutes.

6. Meanwhile, use a deep skillet or wok to heat the olive oil for about half a minute.

7. Caramelize the onion for approximately 5 minutes while frequently tossing. Then combine the garlic and ginger in the pan and heat for another half minute. Keep tossing the pan.

8. Blend the sliced carrots and bell peppers into the skillet and heat for approximately 4 minutes while continuing to toss.

9. Combine the curry paste and fry for another two minutes.

10. Finally, blend the sugar, kale, coconut milk, and the leftover one-half cup of water to the skillet and integrate well.

11. Heat the pan to a slow simmer and fry for

about 8 minutes while continuing to toss occasionally.

12. Turn the burner off and drizzle with soy sauce and salt.

13. Evenly section the curry into serving dishes and serve immediately.

Helpful Tips:

- In Chapter 7, you will find a healthy recipe for low-sodium soy sauce.

- Optional garnish of chopped parsley can go on top or if you need more punch, add sriracha or red pepper flakes.

- You can substitute any of your favorite vegetables in this recipe and will need about three cups total.

- If you prefer, you can remove the kale from this recipe if you like old-fashioned Thai curry.

Turkey Meatloaf

Total Prep & Cooking Time: 80 minutes

Makes: 4 Helpings

Sodium: 197 mg

Protein: 7 gm

Fat: 8 gm

Sugar: 2 gm

Calories: 304

What you need:

For the meatloaf:

- Two oz. carrots, chopped
- One-fourth tsp. lemon zest
- Three-fourths cup vegetable stock, low-salt (See Helpful Tip below)
- Two oz. celery, chopped
- One-half tbsp. vinegar, balsamic

- One-half tsp. ground chili powder, salt-free
- Sixteen oz. turkey, ground
- One-third cup oatmeal, steel-cut
- Two oz. onion, chopped
- One and one-half tbsp. olive oil
- One large egg white
- One-fourth tbsp. garlic, crushed
- olive oil cooking spray

For the sauce:

- Two tbsp. olive oil
- One and one-fourth cups vegetable broth, low-salt (See Helpful Tip below)
- One-half tbsp. garlic, crushed
- Two tbsp. whole wheat flour
- Six oz. mushrooms, sliced
- Two shallots, chopped

Steps:

1. Scrub and thoroughly clean the carrots, celery, mushrooms, and shallots. Chop the vegetables along with the onions and keep them separate and to the side.

2. Adjust the stove temperature to heat at 350° Fahrenheit. Liberally coat a bread pan with the olive oil spray and set to the side.

3. Warm the one and one-half tablespoons of oil in a hot frying pan for about 30 seconds and combine the onions, celery, and carrots. Soften for about 6 minutes.

4. Turn the burner of the stove off and set the skillet to the side.

5. In a big dish, blend the fried vegetables, lemon zest, balsamic vinegar, chili powder, turkey, oatmeal, egg white, and garlic by hand until fully integrated.

6. Transfer the meat to the prepped loaf pan and apply pressure to make sure it is a uniform thickness throughout.

7. Heat in the stove for about 60 minutes.

8. In the meantime, blend the flour and olive oil together thoroughly so there are no lumps

present.

9. Heat the mushrooms, garlic, shallots, and 6 tablespoons of the vegetable stock for approximately 5 minutes.

10. Combine the flour mixture to the skillet and integrate fully while heating for another 60 seconds.

11. Blend the remaining vegetable broth into the pan and reduce for about 10 minutes while the sauce stiffens.

12. Remove from the burner and set to the side.

13. Remove the cooked meatloaf and wait about 10 minutes before dividing into slices and transferring to a serving platter.

14. Empty the sauce over the meatloaf and enjoy immediately.

Helpful Tip:

- See Chapter 7 for the low-sodium vegetable broth recipe to utilize in this recipe.

Veggie Lasagna

Total Prep & Cooking Time: 50 minutes

Makes: 6 Helpings

Sodium: 395 mg

Protein: 10 gm

Fat: 7 gm

Sugar: 6 gm

Calories: 186

What you need:

- One-half cup red bell pepper, diced and separated
- 8 oz. mozzarella cheese, shredded and separated
- Two lasagna noodles, whole wheat and oven-ready
- One and one-half cups marinara sauce, low-sodium and separated (See Helpful Tip

below)
- 8 oz. spinach, chopped and separated
- One-half cup ricotta cheese, low-fat
- 8 oz. mushrooms, sliced and separated

Steps:

1. Prepare the spinach, bell pepper, and mushrooms by properly washing.

2. Chop the spinach and slice the mushrooms. Dice the bell pepper into small sections. Set to the side.

3. Adjust the stove to the temperature of 375° Fahrenheit.

4. Blend two tablespoons of marinara sauce with the ricotta cheese.

5. Cover the base of a 9 x 5-inch glass oven dish with one-third cup of the marinara sauce.

6. Transfer one lasagna noodle over the sauce and layer with another one-third cup of the marinara sauce, one-half cup each of the spinach and mushrooms and one-fourth cup of the bell peppers.

7. Empty the ricotta cheese and evenly

distribute across the pan.

8. Dust the top with a three-fourths cup of the mozzarella cheese.

9. Layer the leftover one-half cup of mushrooms, one-fourth cup of bell peppers, one-half cup of spinach and one-third cup of the marinara sauce.

10. Place the last noodle on top of the sauce.

11. Finish the lasagna by dusting with the remaining marinara sauce and the last one-fourth cup of mozzarella cheese.

12. Layer a section of foil over the pan and heat in the stove for 25 minutes.

13. Take off the tin foil and heat for another 5 minutes and take the pan out of the stove.

14. Wait for 10 minutes before slicing and serving hot. Enjoy!

Helpful Tip:

- Find the recipe for low-sodium marinara sauce in Chapter 7.

Vegetarian Chili

Total Prep & Cooking Time: 55 minutes

Makes: 4 Helpings

Sodium: 443 mg

Protein: 16 gm

Fat: 2 gm

Sugar: 0 gm

Calories: 275

What you need:

- One-fourth medium onion, chopped
- Two cloves garlic, minced
- 14 oz. diced tomatoes, low-sodium with juice
- Three tsp. water
- One-half green bell pepper, diced finely
- Three tsp. soy sauce, low-sodium (See Helpful Tip below)

- One-half red bell pepper, diced finely
- 7.5 oz. can kidney beans, low-sodium and undrained
- One-fourth cup corn
- One-fourth tsp. cayenne pepper
- Six oz. can tomato juice, low-sodium
- One-fourth tsp. oregano seasoning
- One-half tbsp. chili powder, salt-free
- One-fourth tsp. salt
- One-half jalapeno, minced
- Two tbsp. olive oil
- One medium carrot, sliced thinly

Steps:

1. Prepare the carrot and bell peppers by washing thoroughly. Cut the carrot into thin slices and dice the bell peppers. Set to the side.
2. Take the skin off of the onion and roughly chop. Set to the side.

3. Finally, finely chop the jalapeno and set aside.

4. Empty the olive oil into a stockpot and combine the garlic and onion.

5. Heat for approximately 5 minutes and blend the sliced carrots and water. Continue to warm from another 4 minutes.

6. Combine the soy sauce and bell peppers and heat for another two minutes.

7. Turn the burner of the stove down to low.

8. Combine the oregano, salt, kidney beans with the juice, corn, diced tomatoes with the juice, cayenne pepper, tomato juice, and the chili powder and blend until incorporated.

9. Cover and heat for approximately half an hour until properly reduced.

10. Remove from heat and spoon into individual dishes.

11. Serve immediately and enjoy!

Helpful Tip:

- An alternative healthy low-sodium recipe for soy sauce is located in Chapter 7.

Vegetarian Pizza

Total Prep & Cooking Time: 35 minutes

Makes: 4 Slices

Sodium: 479 mg

Protein: 19 gm

Fat: 13 gm

Sugar: 1 gm

Calories: 445

What you need:

- One-third lb. cheese of your choice
- 6 oz. can tomato paste, low-sodium (See Helpful Tips below)
- One 12-inch prepackaged whole wheat pizza crust
- Toppings of your choice

Steps:

1. Set the temperature of the stove to heat at 350° Fahrenheit.
2. Prepare the toppings of your choice by chopping if necessary.
3. Use a pizza stone or pan to lay your crust.
4. Evenly distribute the tomato paste to the edges of the crust.
5. Sprinkle the cheese over the sauce evenly.
6. Arrange the toppings as you desire on top of the cheese.
7. Heat in the stove for approximately 18 minutes and remove.
8. Wait about 10 minutes before slicing and serving. Enjoy!

Helpful Tips:

- Good spices to consider to add extra flavor are basil, garlic powder, parsley, and/or oregano. You can use fresh or dried, whichever your preference.

- If you do want to add meat to this pizza, make sure that it is cooked fully before adding and layer on top of the tomato paste.

- You can use the healthy low-sodium marinara sauce recipe in place of the tomato paste. It is found in Chapter 7.

Zesty Mushroom Soup

Total Prep & Cooking Time: 70 minutes

Makes: 4 Helpings

Sodium: 498 mg

Protein: 21 gm

Fat: 6 gm

Sugar: 1 gm

Calories: 199

What you need:

- One scallion, sliced finely
- One-half tsp. black pepper
- 7 oz. chicken breast
- One-fourth cup white vinegar
- 12 shiitake mushrooms, dried
- One-half cup wood ear mushrooms, chopped
- 8 One-fourth cups water, separated
- One tsp. red pepper flakes
- Three tsp. soy sauce, low-sodium (See Helpful Tips below)
- Two large eggs
- One tsp. ginger, grated finely
- 6 cups chicken broth, low-sodium (See Helpful Tips below)
- One-fourth cup cornstarch
- One tsp. sesame oil
- 4 oz. tofu, firm and cubed
- One tsp. sugar, granulated
- One/eight tsp. salt

Steps:

1. Prepare the scallion and mushrooms by cleaning well and remove any dirt. Chop the scallion into thin slices and roughly chop the wood ear mushrooms and set to the side.
2. In a deep pot, empty 8 cups of the water and heat until boiling. Turn the burner off.
3. Transfer the shiitake mushrooms to the pot and leave to the side for approximately half an hour.
4. Remove the shiitake mushrooms with a slotted spoon and dry thoroughly. Empty the liquid and discard or you may keep for other recipes if you wish.
5. Thinly slice the shiitake mushrooms and set to the side.
6. Using the same pot, blend the soy sauce, chicken broth, sugar, ginger, and sesame oil and allow to come to a slow boil.
7. Transfer the chicken breast to the pot and place a cover on top. Heat for 10 minutes and separate the chicken with the spoon with holes to a plate. Set to the side.

8. After about 5 minutes, take out the bone and shred the meat. Distribute back into the pot.

9. Blend the tofu, wood ear mushrooms, sliced shiitake mushrooms, and vinegar and heat for 10 minutes.

10. Use a glass dish to combine the leftover one-fourth cup of the water and cornstarch until thoroughly combined.

11. Stir the soup while emptying the cornstarch into the pot to integrate fully.

12. In a separate dish, whip the eggs completely.

13. As the soup begins to froth, carefully empty the eggs to flow thinly into the pot while constantly stirring to create small whips.

14. Finally, combine the sliced scallion and transfer to serving bowls.

15. Enjoy immediately!

Helpful Tips:

- If dried shiitake or wood ear mushrooms are not available, you can substitute cremini or Swiss Brown mushrooms in their place.

- To add variety to this soup, you can leave out the chicken breast altogether or substitute shrimp or a white fish in its place.

- You will find healthy recipes for the soy sauce and the chicken broth in Chapter 7.

Chapter 7: Dressings, Sauces & Condiments

Avocado Dressing

Total Prep & Cooking Time: 5 minutes

Makes: 4 Helpings

Sodium: 27 mg

Protein: 1 gm

Fat: 33 gm

Sugar: 0 gm

Calories: 299

What you need:

- Three-fourths tbsp. lemon juice
- 4 oz. olive oil
- 8 oz. avocado
- One/eight tsp. garlic powder

- One-third cup water

Steps:

1. Remove the skin from the avocado and transfer to a food blender.
2. Combine the lemon juice, garlic powder, water, and olive oil to the blender and pulse for approximately 45 seconds until incorporated.
3. Keep in a jar or lidded tub in the fridge for up to 7 days.

Barbeque Sauce

Total Prep & Cooking Time: 90 minutes

Makes: 4 Helpings

Sodium: 38 mg

Protein: 0 gm

Fat: 0 gm

Sugar: 11 gm

Calories: 48

What you need:

- Two-thirds tsp. black pepper
- One tsp. lemon juice
- Two-thirds cup tomato sauce, salt-free (See Helpful Tip below)
- One-third cup water
- Two and two-thirds tbsp. brown sugar
- One and two-thirds tbsp. sugar, granulated

- Two-thirds tsp. ground mustard
- One-third cup apple cider vinegar
- One tsp. Worcestershire sauce, low-sodium (See Helpful Tip below)
- Two-thirds tsp. onion powder

Steps:

1. In a saucepan, blend the tomato sauce, apple cider vinegar, brown sugar, granulated sugar, and water.
2. Season with the pepper, lemon juice, onion powder, mustard, and Worchester shire sauce.
3. Heat the mixture to a slow bubble and turn the temperature of the burner down to the lowest setting.
4. Cover the saucepan and heat for approximately 60 minutes as the sauce reduces.
5. Take the sauce away from the burner and let it rest for a minimum of half an hour before storing in a lidded jar or tub.

Helpful Tip:

- You can use the low-sodium Worcestershire sauce and marinara sauce that is found in this chapter for this recipe.

Chicken Broth

Total Prep & Cooking Time: 2 hours 15 minutes

Makes: 4 cups

Sodium: 42 mg

Protein: 0 gm

Fat: 0 gm

Sugar: 0 gm

Calories: 8

What you need:

- One roasted chicken carcass
- water
- One cup vegetable trimmings, chopped roughly
- Three tbsp. white vinegar

Steps:

1. Use a deep pot to place the chicken carcasses, vinegar, and vegetable scraps.
2. Cover the chicken fully with water and heat until bubbling.
3. Turn the burner down and allow to simmer for approximately 2 hours as the broth reduces.
4. Remove the solid materials with a slotted spoon or tongs. You may also use a fine-mesh strainer if you want purer broth.
5. Place the turkey breast slice on a plate and cover with a thin layer of cream cheese.
6. Transfer to ziplock bags or a lidded tub to store in the freezer for up to a month or can be used immediately.

French Dressing

Total Prep & Cooking Time: 5 minutes

Makes: 4 Helpings

Sodium: 17 mg

Protein: 0 gm

Fat: 6 gm

Sugar: 2 gm

Calories: 56

What you need:

- One/eight cup vinegar, white wine
- One-third tsp. mustard (See Helpful Tip below)
- One/eight cup olive oil
- One-third tsp. tomato paste, low-sodium (See Helpful Tip below)
- One/eight tsp. onion powder
- One-third tsp. honey

Steps:

1. Use a food blender to pulse the mustard, onion powder, tomato paste, olive oil, honey, and vinegar for approximately half a minute.

2. Remove to a lidded tub or Mason jar to store in the fridge. It will keep for about two weeks.

Helpful Tip:

- Look for the alternative recipe for low-sodium mustard and marinara sauce located in this chapter.

Italian Dressing

Total Prep & Cooking Time: 5 minutes

Makes: 4 Helpings (One tablespoon per helping)

Sodium: 14 mg

Protein: 0 gm

Fat: 13 gm

Sugar: 1 gm

Calories: 119

What you need:

- One tsp. sugar, granulated
- Two oz. olive oil
- One oz. vinegar, white wine
- One and one-half tbsp. water
- One tsp. basil seasoning
- Three-fourths tsp. Mrs. Dash's seasoning mix
- One-half tbsp. mayonnaise, low-sodium

(See Helpful Tip below)
- One-fourth tsp. garlic powder

Steps:

1. Use a food blender to pulse the vinegar, olive oil, mayonnaise, sugar, and water for about 15 seconds.
2. Combine the garlic powder, basil, and Mrs. Dash into the blender and pulse for an additional 30 seconds until smooth.
3. Transfer to a glass container or tub that has a cover and refrigerate for 5 days until needed.

Helpful Tips:

- There is a healthy mayonnaise recipe low in sodium located in Chapter 7.

Ketchup

Total Prep & Cooking Time: 5 minutes

Makes: 10 Helpings (One Tablespoon per helping)

Sodium: 24 mg

Protein: 0 gm

Fat: 0 gm

Sugar: 2 gm

Calories: 15

What you need:

- One tbsp. honey
- One-half tsp. garlic powder
- Three oz. tomato paste, salt-free (See Helpful Tip below)
- One oz. cup water
- One-half tsp. onion powder
- One-fourth tsp. salt
- One and one-half tsp. mustard (See

Helpful Tip below)

- One oz. white wine vinegar

Steps:

1. Use a blender to pulse the tomato paste, onion powder, vinegar, garlic powder, honey, salt, mustard, and water for approximately 30 seconds until thoroughly combined.

2. Distribute to a Mason jar or lidded container to keep in the fridge for up to 14 days.

Helpful Tip:

- There is a low-sodium alternative recipe for mustard and marinara sauce in this chapter.

Marinara Sauce

Total Prep & Cooking Time: 75 minutes

Makes: 4 Helpings

Sodium: 21 mg

Protein: 2 gm

Fat: 0 gm

Sugar: 7 gm

Calories: 52

What you need:

- Three-fourths tbsp. sugar, granulated
- One/eight cup onions, chopped
- 8 oz. can tomato sauce, salt-free (See Helpful Tip below)
- Three-fourths tbsp. ground oregano seasoning

- 4 tbsp. tomato paste, salt-free (See Helpful Tip below)
- One and one-half tbsp. garlic, minced
- olive oil cooking spray
- One tbsp. basil seasoning
- Three-fourths cups water
- One/eight tsp. red pepper flakes, crushed

Steps:

1. Remove the outer skin from the onion and chop into small cubes.
2. Coat a skillet with the olive oil spray, empty the onions and brown for approximately 5 minutes.
3. Blend the water, tomato paste, and sauce into the frying pan and toss to completely coat the onions.
4. Season with the oregano, garlic, sugar, basil, and red pepper flakes and blend until combined.
5. Turn the burner to low and simmer for

approximately half an hour.

6. Take away from the burner and cool for another half hour before storing.

Helpful Tip:

- You can use the healthy low-sodium marinara sauce recipe in place of the tomato paste and sauce. It is found in Chapter 7.

Mayonnaise

Total Prep & Cooking Time: 10 minutes

Makes: 8 Helpings (One tablespoon per helping)

Sodium: 50 mg

Protein: 0 gm

Fat: 9 gm

Sugar: 0 gm

Calories: 84

What you need:

- One/eight tsp. black pepper
- Three and one/eight cups tepid water
- One/eight tsp. salt
- Two cups ice water
- Three-fourths tbsp. lemon juice
- One large egg yolk
- One-third cup olive oil

Steps:

1. Blend the egg yolk, lemon juice, and three-fourths tablespoons of the water to a metal dish.
2. Heat the remaining tepid water in a saucepan until bubbling.
3. Empty the ice cubes into another dish and set to the side.
4. When the water begins to steam, move the egg bowl over the saucepan and continuously whip the mixture until it thickens.
5. Transfer the meal to the dish with the ice water and stir continuously for two additional minutes.
6. Empty the dish into a food blender and combine the pepper, olive oil, and salt while pulsing for approximately 90 seconds until it thickens properly.
7. Store in a glass container or a tub with a cover in the fridge for a maximum of a week.

Mustard

Total Prep & Cooking Time: Two0 minutes

Makes: 24 Helpings (One tablespoon per helping)

Sodium: 74 mg

Protein: 1 gm

Fat: 1 gm

Sugar: 0 gm

Calories: 16

What you need:

- One-third cup apple cider vinegar
- Three-fourths tsp. salt
- One-fourth tsp. turmeric seasoning
- One-half cup ground mustard
- One-fourth tsp. garlic powder
- One-half cup water
- One/eight tsp. paprika seasoning

Steps:

1. Blend the salt, ground mustard, garlic powder, turmeric, and paprika in a saucepan until incorporated.

2. Combine the apple cider vinegar and water into the pan and blend well.

3. Heat until it bubbles and adjust the temperature of the burner to the lowest setting. Continue to heat for approximately 8 minutes while making sure to keep stirring the pot.

4. As it thickens, remove from the burner and set to the side for about 60 seconds.

5. Use a lid to cover the saucepan and keep off the heat for approximately 15 minutes.

6. Transfer to a lidded tub or glass mason jars once completely cooled and keep in the refrigerator for about three days.

Peanut Butter

Total Prep & Cooking Time: 10 minutes

Makes: 4 Helpings

Sodium: 18 mg

Protein: 16 gm

Fat: 7 gm

Sugar: 2 gm

Calories: 190

What you need:

- One/eight tsp. salt
- One cup roasted peanuts, unsalted
- Two tsp. sugar, granulated
- One-fourth tbsp. olive oil

Steps:

1. Use a food blender to pulse the olive oil, roasted peanuts, sugar, and salt together for approximately 10 minutes.

2. Use a rubber scraper to remove the peanut butter from the sides of the dish as needed as it becomes smoother.

3. Transfer to a mason jar or a tub with a cover and keep fresh in the refrigerator up to one month.

Ranch Dressing

Total Prep & Cooking Time: 5 minutes

Makes: 8 Helpings (One tablespoon per helping)

Sodium: 17 mg

Protein: 0 gm

Fat: 0 gm

Sugar: 1 gm

Calories: 8

What you need:

- One/eight cup sour cream, fat-free
- One-fourth cup buttermilk, low-fat
- One/eight tsp. black pepper
- One-fourth tbsp. dill weed, chopped
- One/eight tsp. garlic powder
- One-fourth tbsp. parsley, chopped
- One-fourth tbsp. mustard, low-sodium (See Helpful Tip below)

- One-fourth tsp. onion powder

Steps:

1. Use a big glass dish to blend the buttermilk, sour cream, and mustard until integrated.
2. Season with the dill weed, pepper, parsley, garlic powder, and onion powder until combined.
3. Transfer to a glass jar or lidded tub to store in refrigerator up to 7 days.

Helpful Tip:

- Find the low-sodium healthy mustard recipe located in Chapter 7.

Soy Sauce

Total Prep & Cooking Time: 70 minutes

Makes: 4 Helpings

Sodium: 25 mg

Protein: 0 gm

Fat: 1 gm

Sugar: 0 gm

Calories: 23

What you need:

- Two tsp. brown sugar
- One tsp. vinegar, balsamic
- Two tbsp. vegetable broth, low-salt (See Helpful Tips below)
- One-fourth tsp. black pepper
- One tsp. sesame oil
- One/eight tsp. garlic powder
- Three tsp. vinegar, red wine

- Two oz. water

Steps:

1. Warm the water in a saucepan until it is bubbling. Turn the burner off.
2. Blend the vinegars, vegetable broth, sesame oil, garlic powder, brown sugar, and pepper and fully combine.
3. Wait approximately 60 minutes before serving.

Helpful Tips:

- Use the low-sodium recipe for vegetable broth located in this chapter.

- This sauce can be stored up to 30 days in the fridge in a sealed jar.

Taco Seasoning

Total Prep & Cooking Time: 5 minutes

Makes: One Packet of Taco Seasoning (7 teaspoons)

Sodium: 148 mg

Protein: 2 gm

Fat: 3 gm

Sugar: 1 gm

Calories: 59

What you need:

- Three-fourths tbsp. cornstarch
- One-fourth cup chili powder, salt-free
- Three-fourths tbsp. paprika seasoning
- One-fourth tbsp. onion powder
- One/eight cup cumin seasoning
- One-fourth tbsp. garlic powder

Steps:

1. Use a mason jar to shake the chili powder, cumin, paprika, garlic powder, cornstarch, and onion powder until thoroughly combined.
2. Store in the pantry or on the countertop.

Tartar Sauce

Total Prep & Cooking Time: 5 minutes

Makes: 10 Helpings (One Tablespoon per helping)

Sodium: 58 mg

Protein: 0 gm

Fat: 3 gm

Sugar: 0 gm

Calories: 33

What you need:

- One-half cup mayonnaise, low-sodium (See Helpful Tip below)
- Three tsp. onion, minced
- One-half tsp. lemon juice
- One and one-half tsp. sugar, granulated
- Three tsp. sweet relish, low-sodium

Steps:

1. Use a food blender to pulse the sugar, mayonnaise, lemon juice, onion and relish for approximately half a minute until incorporated.
2. Transfer into a lidded tub or Mason jar and keep fresh in the fridge for 7 days.

Helpful Tip:

- Look for the alternative healthy low-sodium recipe for mayonnaise located in this chapter.

Thai Marinade

Total Prep & Cooking Time: 5 minutes

Makes: 4 Helpings

Sodium: 6 mg

Protein: 1 gm

Fat: 0 gm

Sugar: 1 gm

Calories: 11

What you need:

- Three cloves garlic, minced
- One tsp. red pepper flakes
- Two oz. lime juice
- One-fourth cup parsley seasoning
- Two oz. lemon juice
- One-half tsp. ginger seasoning

Steps:

1. Use a food blender to pulse the red pepper flakes, lemon juice, ginger, lime juice, parsley, and garlic for about half a minute.

2. Transfer to a ziplock bag or lidded container and keep fresh in the refrigerator for 5 days or freeze for 30 days.

Thousand Island Dressing

Total Prep & Cooking Time: 5 minutes

Makes: 4 Helpings (One tablespoon per helping)

Sodium: 19 mg

Protein: 0 gm

Fat: 0 gm

Sugar: 2 gm

Calories: 15

What you need:

- One/eight cups yogurt, no-fat and plain
- One-fourth tsp. vinegar, white
- Two-thirds tbsp. ketchup, salt-free (See Helpful Tip below)
- One-third tsp. white onion, chopped finely
- One tsp. sweet relish, low-sodium
- One-fourth tsp. sugar, granulated
- One/eight tsp. black pepper

Steps:

1. Use a food blender to combine the yogurt, vinegar, ketchup, chopped onion, and relish for approximately half a minute.
2. Blend the sugar and pepper into the mixture for another 15 seconds and transfer to a lidded container or a glass jar to keep in the fridge for up to 14 days.

Helpful Tip:

- Located in this chapter is an alternative low-sodium recipe for ketchup.

Tzatziki Sauce

Total Prep & Cooking Time: 5 minutes

Makes: 4 Helpings

Sodium: 159 mg

Protein: 3 gm

Fat: 4 gm

Sugar: 1 gm

Calories: 56

What you need:

- Three tsp. dill, chopped
- One clove garlic, minced
- One-fourth tsp. salt
- Three tsp. olive oil
- One-half tsp. lemon zest
- 4 oz. Greek yogurt, plain
- Three tsp. lemon juice

Steps:

1. Use a blender to pulse the Greek yogurt, lemon zest, lemon juice, salt, olive oil, garlic, and dill for approximately half a minute and remove.
2. Keep in a lidded tub or jar for up to two weeks in the fridge.

Vegetable Broth

Total Prep & Cooking Time: 75 minutes

Makes: 5 cups

Sodium: 35 mg

Protein: 0 gm

Fat: 0 gm

Sugar: 0 gm

Calories: 5

What you need:

- One-third clove garlic including skin, chopped roughly
- One-fourth cup saved vegetable scraps (See Helpful Tips below)
- One/eight onion including skin, chopped roughly
- One-fourth carrots including skin, chopped finely

- One-third stalk celery, chopped
- One and one-half oz. tomatoes, chopped roughly
- One/eight tsp. peppercorns, whole
- Three-fourths oz. mixed greens, chopped roughly
- One-third sprig thyme
- One and one/eighth sprigs parsley, chopped roughly
- One/eight tsp. salt
- water
- One-third bay leaf

Steps:

1. Use a deep pot to combine all the listed materials and ensure the vegetable scraps are fully covered with water.
2. Heat the broth until bubbling and then put the temperature of the burner down to low.
3. Place a cover on the pot and lightly heat for approximately 60 minutes.
4. Remove from the heat for about 20 minutes.
5. Use a strainer with fine-mesh to remove

the solids and store in a lidded tub or ziplock bag in the refrigerator for 5 days. It will keep up to 30 days in the freezer.

Helpful Tips:

- While you are making your meals for the week, save any scraps from the vegetable dishes that you would otherwise discard. These vegetables would include bell peppers, mushrooms, lettuce, garlic, scallions, celery, carrots, and onions.

- If you plan on making this recipe within a week, simply put these scraps in a zipping plastic storage bag and keep refrigerated until ready to use. Any time longer, you can easily freeze them.

- To add more flavoring to your vegetable broth, add one large potato chopped roughly and/or one-fourth cup of mushrooms that are chopped roughly.

Worcestershire Sauce

Total Prep & Cooking Time: 15 minutes

Makes: 20 Helpings (One tablespoon per helping)

Sodium: 58 mg

Protein: 0 gm

Fat: 3 gm

Sugar: 0 gm

Calories: 33

What you need:

- One-third tsp. black pepper
- One/eight tsp. ground clove
- One-third cup tomato paste, salt-free (See Helpful Tip below)
- One/eight cup shallots, chopped finely
- One-third cup cider vinegar
- Three-fourths tbsp. maple syrup
- One-third tsp. cardamom seasoning

- One/eight tsp. chili powder, salt-free
- One-third tsp. ground ginger
- One/eight cup honey
- One-third tsp. olive oil
- One/eight tsp. ground cinnamon

Steps:

1. Warm the olive oil in a pan for about half a minute. Fry the shallots for approximately 8 minutes.
2. Lower the burner temperature to low and blend the tomato sauce in the frying pan. Heat for approximately two minutes and take the skillet away from the burner.
3. Combine the ground cinnamon, cider vinegar, ground clove, cardamom, maple syrup, ginger, chili powder, and pepper into the pan and incorporate fully.
4. Leave the pan to sit for approximately 10 minutes and empty the contents into a food blender along with the honey.
5. Pulse for approximately 45 seconds.
6. Use a fine-mesh strainer to withdraw and

separate the solid materials and transfer the Worcestershire sauce in a Mason jar or lidded tub to store in the refrigerator up to a month.

Helpful Tip:

- You can use the healthy low-sodium marinara sauce recipe in place of the tomato paste. It is found in Chapter 7.

Yogurt Dressing

Total Prep & Cooking Time: 5 minutes

Makes: 4 Helpings

Sodium: 4 mg

Protein: 13 gm

Fat: 4 gm

Sugar: 18 gm

Calories: 192

What you need:

- Two tsp. lemon zest
- 4 cloves garlic
- 10.5 oz. natural yogurt, low-fat
- Two tsp. black pepper
- 6 tsp. mint
- 4 tbsp. lemon juice

Steps:

1. Use a glass dish to combine the garlic, yogurt, pepper, lemon juice, lemon zest, and mint until integrated completely.

2. Keep fresh in the fridge for a maximum of a week or serve immediately.

Chapter 8: Snacks and Desserts

Apple Crumb Cake Muffins

Total Prep & Cooking Time: 45 minutes

Makes: 12 Muffins

Sodium: 110 mg

Protein: 2 gm

Fat: 12 gm

Sugar: 6 gm

Calories: 225

What you need:

For the apples:

- One/eight tsp. ground cinnamon
- One and one-third tsp. sugar, granulated
- One-half cup of water
- One and two-thirds cups apples

For the topping:

- One/eight tsp. salt
- One-third cup whole wheat flour
- Two tbsp. margarine, unsalted
- One-third cup brown sugar

For the batter:

- Two-thirds tsp. baking soda
- One large egg
- Two-thirds tsp. vinegar, white
- One/eight tsp. salt
- Two-thirds tsp. ground cinnamon

- One-third cup olive oil
- Two-thirds cup sugar, granulated
- One and one-third cups whole wheat flour
- Two-thirds cup sour cream, low-fat
- Two tsp. vanilla extract

Steps:

1. Adjust the temperature of the stove to heat at 350° Fahrenheit. Use silicone or baking cups to line a cupcake pan and set to the side.

2. Prepare the apples by taking off the skin with a knife or peeler. Core to take out the seeds and chop into small cubes.

3. Use a microwave-safe dish to empty the apples and water and nuke for approximately two minutes until softened.

4. Withdraw the water from the dish and dust with the cinnamon and sugar. Set aside.

5. Use a saucepan to dissolve the margarine completely. Empty into a glass dish and blend with the flour, brown sugar, and salt. Set to the side.

6. In a food blender, pulse the olive oil,

sugar, salt, cinnamon, baking soda, vinegar, and vanilla extract for approximately 60 seconds until combined.

7. Blend the flour and sour cream into the batter for another half minute.

8. Use a rubber scraper to integrate the cooked apples, fully coating them in the batter.

9. Evenly distribute the batter to the prepped cupcake tin to approximately two-thirds full.

10. Spoon the apple crumble over the top of each muffin cup.

11. Heat in the stove for about 17 minutes and remove from the oven.

12. Move the cupcakes to a wire rack and wait about 10 minutes before serving.

Carrot Dip

Total Prep & Cooking Time: 30 minutes

Makes: 4 Helpings

Sodium: 101 mg

Protein: 5 gm

Fat: 3 gm

Sugar: 4 gm

Calories: 76

What you need:

- One-third tsp. harissa
- One tsp. cumin seasoning
- One/eight cup Greek yogurt, low-fat
- 6 oz. carrots
- One tsp. olive oil
- One/eight cup feta cheese, crumbled
- One tsp. olives

Steps:

1. Adjust your stove to broil. Cover a flat pan that has a rim with foil.
2. Thoroughly scrub the carrots and slice diagonally into two-inch sections. Transfer to the prepped sheet.
3. Distribute the olive oil over the carrots and dust with the cumin.
4. Heat in the stove for approximately 20 minutes and remove.
5. Use a food blender and the combine the carrots, Greek yogurt, and harissa for approximately two minutes until smooth.
6. Distribute to a bowl and garnish with the olives and feta cheese and enjoy immediately.

Cauliflower Rice

Total Prep & Cooking Time: 15 minutes

Makes: 4 Helpings

Sodium: 20 mg

Protein: 1 gm

Fat: 3 gm

Sugar: 2 gm

Calories: 46

What you need:

- One clove garlic, minced
- Three tsp. olive oil
- One small head cauliflower, cut into florets
- One-half tsp. salt

Steps:

1. Remove the stem of the cauliflower and wash well.

2. Use a food blender to pulse the cauliflower for approximately two minutes until the consistency is crumbly.

3. Warm the olive oil in a frying pan and heat the garlic for about 60 seconds.

4. Combine the riced cauliflower and heat for approximately 8 minutes while occasionally tossing.

5. Remove from the burner and serve immediately.

Helpful Tip:

- This recipe is a good alternative for brown rice for any dish or as a side.

Fiesta Dip

Total Prep & Cooking Time: 35 minutes

Makes: 8 Helpings

Sodium: 340 mg

Protein: 8 gm

Fat: 1 gm

Sugar: 6 gm

Calories: 134

What you need:

- Four cups lettuce, shredded
- Eight oz. can black beans, low-sodium
- One cup onion, diced
- Two cups cherry tomatoes, chopped and separated
- Four oz. roasted red peppers, chopped

- Three One-half tsp. taco seasoning, separated (See Helpful Tip below)
- Four oz. turkey, ground
- One oz. cheddar cheese, shredded
- Three tbsp. olive oil
- Four oz. sour cream, low-fat
- Two One-half cups butternut squash

Steps:

1. Thoroughly wash the lettuce, butternut squash, and tomatoes. Chop the lettuce and set to the side.

2. Slice the butternut squash into small cubes and transfer to a microwave-safe container.

3. Remove the skin of the onion and chop into small pieces and transfer to a glass dish. Chop the tomatoes and combine one cup with the onions. Set aside.

4. Empty two tablespoons of the water in the squash container and heat in the microwave for approximately 6 minutes.

5. In the meantime, use a saucepan to heat the beans for about 5 minutes and turn the burner of the stove off. Set the pan to the side.

6. Use oven mitts to remove the container and crush the squash fully with a masher. Blend one and one-half teaspoons of the taco seasoning until completely combined. Set to the side.

7. Warm the oil in a hot frying pan and blend the ground turkey, the remaining two teaspoons of taco seasoning, and the remaining cup of tomatoes.

8. Use a wooden spatula to break the meat into smaller chunks and heat for approximately 8 minutes until browned.

9. In a big serving dish, layer the lettuce, mashed squash, onions, sour cream, beans, and the meat.

10. Top with the cheese and red peppers and serve immediately.

Helpful Tip:

- Use the healthy low-sodium taco seasoning found in Chapter 7.

Macaroni & Cheese

Total Prep & Cooking Time: 30 minutes

Makes: 4 Helpings

Sodium: 418 mg

Protein: 7 gm

Fat: 41 gm

Sugar: 8 gm

Calories: 503

What you need:

- One tsp. black pepper, separated
- Three tbsp. olive oil, separated
- One and one-half tsp. ground mustard
- 30 oz. can light coconut milk
- Two medium heads cauliflower
- One-half tsp. garlic salt
- 4 oz. carrots
- One-half cup whole wheat flour

- Two tbsp. margarine
- One-half tsp. salt
- Three tsp. onion powder

Steps:

1. Dissolve one tablespoon of the olive oil in a soup pot. Combine one-half teaspoon of the pepper, garlic, salt, and flour and heat for approximately half a minute.
2. Empty the mixture into a bowl and keep to the side.
3. Thoroughly wash the cauliflower and carrots. Dice the carrots into small sections.
4. Remove the stem and chop the cauliflower into half-inch strips and transfer to the pot.
5. Combine the salt, ground mustard, onion powder, the remaining two tablespoons of olive oil, margarine, coconut milk, carrots, and the remaining one-half teaspoon of the pepper into the pot.
6. Use a cover and warm for approximately

10 minutes.

7. As the mixture starts to boil, take the lid off and reduce for another 10 minutes.

8. Spoon onto individual plates and dust with the flour mixture.

9. Immediately serve while still hot and enjoy!

Mozzarella Sticks

Total Prep & Cooking Time: 80 minutes

Makes: 4 Helpings (4 sticks per helping)

Sodium: 395 mg

Protein: 15 gm

Fat: 7 gm

Sugar: 0 gm

Calories: 157

What you need:

- Three One-third tbsp. panko breadcrumbs
- One large egg
- One and one-third tbsp. whole wheat flour
- 8 sticks of string cheese, low-sodium
- One and one-third tbsp. parmesan cheese
- olive oil cooking spray

Steps:

1. Chop the cheese sticks into halves and set in the freezer for approximately 60 minutes.

2. About 10 minutes before you are ready to proceed, adjust the temperature of the stove to 400° Fahrenheit. Cover a flat sheet with foil and set to the side.

3. Set out three glass dishes and empty the breadcrumbs and parmesan cheese into one, flour into the second, and whip the egg in the other.

4. Remove the frozen cheese from the freezer.

5. Use a fork to immerse one piece of cheese into the flour, the egg, and then the breadcrumbs. Transfer to the prepped sheet.

6. Repeat step 5 for all the cheese until complete.

7. Coat the sticks with olive oil spray and heat for approximately 4 minutes.

8. Remove and enjoy immediately!

Helpful Tip:

- Couple this recipe with the marinara dipping sauce that is found in Chapter 7.

Peanut Butter Bars

Total Prep & Cooking Time: 4 hours 15 minutes

Makes: 12 Bars

Sodium: 62 mg

Protein: 9 gm

Fat: 24 gm

Sugar: 1 gm

Calories: 299

What you need:

For the batter:

- One-fourth tsp. salt
- Two tbsp. margarine
- One cup whole wheat flour
- One-third tsp. vanilla extract

For the peanut butter layer:

- One cup whole wheat flour, separated
- 12 oz. peanut butter, creamy and unsalted (See Helpful Tip below)
- Two-thirds cup sugar, granulated and separated
- One-fourth tsp. salt
- Three-fourths tsp. vanilla extract

For the topping:

- Three tbsp. baking chocolate,

unsweetened
- One and one-half tsp. margarine
- Three tbsp. sugar, confectioner
- One and one-half tbsp. roasted peanuts, unsalted and crushed
- One-fourth tsp. vanilla extract

Steps:

1. Dissolve the butter in a saucepan and combine in a glass dish with the flour, salt and vanilla extract until blended.
2. Layer an 8-inch pan with baking lining and apply pressure to evenly distribute the batter into the base. Move to the fridge to set for approximately 5 minutes.
3. In the meantime, use another dish to combine a one-half cup of the flour, peanut butter, vanilla extract, salt, and sugar and integrate fully.
4. Transfer from the pan to the fridge and distribute the peanut butter across the pan evenly using a rubber scraper.
5. Use the same saucepan to liquefy the

chocolate and the butter while occasionally stirring.

6. Blend the sugar and vanilla extract in the chocolate and incorporate fully.

7. Empty the chocolate over the pan evenly.

8. Dust the top with the peanuts and refrigerate for approximately 4 hours. Alternatively, you can freeze for 60 minutes.

9. Remove and slice into 12 individual bars and serve immediately.

Helpful Tip:

- Look in Chapter 7 for the healthy alternative low-sodium peanut butter recipe.

Potato Salad

Total Prep & Cooking Time: 60 minutes

Makes: 4 Helpings

Sodium: 32 mg

Protein: 3 gm

Fat: 4 gm

Sugar: 1 gm

Calories: 192

What you need:

- One-half tbsp. olive oil
- Twelve oz. russet potatoes, unpeeled and chopped
- One-half clove garlic, minced
- Two oz. sour cream, fat-free
- One-half tbsp. apple cider vinegar
- One large egg
- Two oz. celery, chopped

- One/eight cup sweet onion, chopped
- Six cups water
- Four cups cold water
- One/eight tsp. black pepper

Steps:

1. Thoroughly scrub the celery and chop the onion and celery. Set to the side.

2. Use a saucepan to empty two cups of the cold water on top of the egg.

3. As the water starts to boil, adjust a timer for 7 minutes.

4. Remove the boiled water and distribute the remaining two cups of cold water on top of the egg. Set to the side to cool.

5. After approximately 5 minutes, take off the shell and chop roughly. Set to the side.

6. In the meantime, use a deep saucepan to arrange the potatoes and insert water to about an inch above the unpeeled potatoes.

7. Warm until the water is bubbling and adjust the burner of the stove to the lowest temperature.

8. Position a lid on the saucepan and warm for another 22 minutes.

9. Withdraw the water from the pan and wait about 5 minutes before dividing into small cubes.

10. Use a glass serving dish to blend the pepper, garlic, vinegar, and olive oil together completely.

11. Combine the onion, celery, sour cream, potatoes, and egg, tossing to apply seasoning throughout.

12. Serve immediately and enjoy!

Red Pepper Hummus

Total Prep & Cooking Time: 35 minutes

Makes: 4 Helpings

Sodium: 544 mg

Protein: 6 gm

Fat: 5 gm

Sugar: 5 gm

Calories: 485

What you need:

- One and one-half cups red peppers
- One clove garlic
- Two-thirds tbsp. water
- One-third tsp. paprika seasoning
- One-half tsp. salt
- Ten oz. can garbanzo beans, low-sodium, drained and washed
- Two-thirds tbsp. olive oil

- One-eight cup lemon juice
- Two-third tsp. cumin seasoning

Steps:

1. Adjust the stove to the setting of broil.
2. Layer a section of foil over a flat sheet.
3. Remove the seeds and middle of the red peppers and position the peppers in one layer on the prepped pan.
4. Heat in the stove for approximately 13 minutes and remove from the heat. Set to the side for about 10 minutes.
5. Portion 1/2 cup of the peppers to the side and transfer the remaining cup of peppers to a food blender.
6. Combine the paprika, cumin, salt, water, olive oil, garlic, lemon juice, and garbanzo beans into the blender and pulse for approximately 2 minutes until creamy.
7. Distribute to a serving dish and garnish with the 1/2 cup of peppers.
8. Serve immediately and enjoy!

Helpful Tip:

- The hummus will stay fresh up to 7 days in the refrigerator when stored in a lidded container.
-
- Other garnishes you can add to this recipe are 1/3 teaspoon of paprika and/or 1/2 tablespoon of olive oil.

Rice Pudding

Total Prep & Cooking Time: 70 minutes

Makes: 4 Helpings

Sodium: 115 mg

Protein: 11 gm

Fat: 6 gm

Sugar: 17 gm

Calories: 290

What you need:

- Two tsp. vanilla extract
- 4 cups milk, skim and divided
- One tsp. ground cinnamon
- One/eight tsp. nutmeg seasoning
- Two tbsp. sugar, granulated
- One cup brown rice, uncooked

Steps:

1. In a deep saucepan, blend the sugar, nutmeg, cinnamon, vanilla extract, rice, and three cups of the skim milk.

2. Warm the pan and as it begins to bubble, adjust the heat of the burner down to low.

3. Use a lid and reduce the pudding for approximately 50 minutes.

4. Take the pan off of the burner and blend in the remaining cup of milk.

5. Immediately serve and enjoy!

South American Guacamole

Total Prep & Cooking Time: 10 minutes

Makes: 4 Helpings

Sodium: 82 mg

Protein: 2 gm

Fat: 10 gm

Sugar: 2 gm

Calories: 113

What you need:

- One avocado, cubed
- One/eight tsp. salt
- 12 sprigs cilantro, chopped
- Three tsp. red onion, chopped
- One large tomato, deseeded and chopped

Steps:

1. Remove the skin from the onion and toss out. Wash the tomato thoroughly.

2. Slice the tomato and remove the seeds. Chop along with the onion and cilantro. Set to the side.

3. Remove the skin from the avocado and slice into large cubes.

4. Blend the avocado, salt, cilantro, red onion, and tomato in a glass dish until combined.

5. Enjoy immediately.

Stuffed Mushrooms

Total Prep & Cooking Time: 30 minutes

Makes: 4 Helpings

Sodium: 321 mg

Protein: 8 gm

Fat: 8 gm

Sugar: 2 gm

Calories: 172

What you need:

For the mushrooms:

- One and one-half tbsp. breadcrumbs
- One-fourth tsp. black pepper
- 8 cremini mushrooms
- One-half tbsp. capers, chopped
- Three tsp. green pepper, diced finely
- olive oil cooking spray

- One and one-half tbsp. walnuts, chopped finely
- Three tsp. onions, diced
- One-fourth tsp. marjoram seasoning
- mushroom stems and meat that was removed
- One-fourth tsp. ground coriander seasoning
- Three tsp. olive oil
- One slice cheddar cheese, fat-free
- One/eight cup dry white wine

For the coating:

- One-fourth cup breadcrumbs
- Two oz. half & half, fat-free
- One-fourth cup whole wheat flour

Steps:

1. Set the stove to heat at the temperature of 400° Fahrenheit.
2. Properly remove any dirt from the mushrooms.
3. Remove the stems and inside meat of the mushrooms with a spoon and set to the side.
4. Set out a cupcake tin and distribute one-third teaspoon of olive oil into 8 of the wells. Set aside.
5. Coat a frying pan with oil spray and combine the walnuts, mushroom meat that was removed earlier, pepper, and onion for about three minutes while occasionally tossing.
6. Blend the breadcrumbs, white wine, capers, green pepper, marjoram, coriander, and pepper into the pan and heat for another 4 minutes while tossing occasionally. Turn the burner off.
7. In the meantime, set out 3 dishes for the flour, half and half, and breadcrumbs.
8. Scoop the filling into each of the mushrooms and evenly distribute the sliced cheese to each.
9. Take one mushroom using a fork and immerse into the flour, half and half, and then

the breadcrumbs. Transfer to the cupcake tin.

10. Repeat for each of the mushrooms until complete.

11. Heat the tin in the stove for 8 minutes. Turn the mushrooms to the other side. Warm from another 3 minutes.

12.   Serve immediately and enjoy!

Tomato Salsa

Total Prep & Cooking Time: 45 minutes

Makes: 4 Helpings

Sodium: 105 mg

Protein: 1 gm

Fat: 2 gm

Sugar: 2 gm

Calories: 35

What you need:

- Three tsp. lime juice
- One-fourth tsp. black pepper
- Three sprigs cilantro
- One Serrano pepper
- olive oil cooking spray
- One-fourth tsp. salt
- One clove garlic
- Two large whole red tomatoes

- One-fourth cup onion
- One-half tbsp. olive oil

Steps:

1. Set your stove to the broil setting. Layer a flat pan with a rim with foil and apply a generous layer of the olive oil spray.

2. Divide the tomatoes into halves and arrange on the prepped sheet with the skin on the foil.

3. Put on a pair of gloves. Section the Serrano pepper into two parts and discard the seeds. Distribute to the foiled pan.

4. Transfer the garlic and onion to the prepped pan.

5. Pour the olive oil on top of the vegetables to coat well.

6. Heat in the stove for approximately 12 minutes until the vegetables start to turn black.

7. Remove from the stove to the counter for about 10 minutes.

8. Use a food blender to pulse the pepper, cooked vegetables, lime juice, salt, and cilantro

for approximately 2 minutes.

9. Serve immediately and enjoy!

Trail Mix

Total Prep & Cooking Time: 5 minutes

Makes: 4 Helpings

Sodium: 1 mg

Protein: 4 gm

Fat: 12 gm

Sugar: 6 gm

Calories: 154

What you need:

- One/eight cup raisins
- One-fourth cup almonds, unsalted
- One/eight cup dark chocolate chips
- One-fourth cup pecan, unsalted and sliced
- One/eight cup pumpkin seeds, shelled and

unsalted

- One-fourth cup apples, dried
- One/eight cup walnuts, shelled and chopped

Steps:

1. Use a lidded container to empty all the ingredients and agitate until fully combined.

2. Can be stored in the pantry or on the countertop for up to two weeks.

Helpful Tip:

- To add variety, you can substitute sunflower seeds or unsalted pretzels in the mix.

Conclusion

The delicious recipes included will ensure you will never get bored with the same meals every day as there is a wide array of meals, snacks, desserts, sauces, and condiments included along with recipe variations. Filling and healthy, all these recipes will keep you focused on your personal weight loss goals of becoming more healthy and staying around longer for your family and friends.

When using this cookbook, you will find the results that you are looking for quickly as it is all laid out in an easy to follow format to help you understand how to incorporate the DASH Diet into your life today and not getting giving up after trying for a week, a common downfall for any new diet.

There are many variations that you can experiment with in the dozens of recipes that you will receive and can work with all the taste preferences for you and the family. You will find the American staples inside as well as International delights that are easy enough to have the kids' help.

Index for the Recipes

Chapter 4: Breakfast Recipes

Bacon Egg & Spinach Casserole
Biscuits & Gravy
Breakfast Tostadas
Creamy Oatmeal
Egg Salad
Eggs Benedict
Fruit Smoothie
Green Smoothie
Homemade Bacon
Oatmeal Pancakes
Sausage Patties
Stuffed Potatoes
Quiche Cups

Chapter 5: Lunch Recipes

American Chopsuey
Asian Chicken Wraps
Baked Chicken
Cheesy Mushroom Risotto
Chicken Gyros
Chicken Salad
Fettuccine Alfredo
Fish Fillets
Fish Stew
Fried Rice
Mexican Salad

Minestrone Soup
Mushroom Fajitas
Orange Chicken
Oven Baked Sea Bass
Quinoa Salad
Sloppy Joe Sandwich
Spaghetti with Vegetables
Tuna Salad
Turkey Panini
Turkey Tacos
Vegetable Soup
Veggie Jambalaya
Zucchini Frittata

Chapter 6: Dinner Recipes

Baked Salmon
Beef Stroganoff
Black Bean Burgers
Chicken Kabobs
Crunchy Fried Chicken
Herbed Oven Roasted Veggies
Lintel Stew
Mashed Potatoes
Pumpkin Soup
Red Beans & Rice
Sesame Chicken
Thai Vegetable Curry
Turkey Meatloaf
Veggie Lasagna
Vegetarian Chili
Vegetarian Pizza

Zesty Mushroom Soup

Chapter 7: Dressings, Sauces & Condiments

Avocado Dressing
Barbeque Sauce
Chicken Broth
French Dressing
Italian Dressing
Ketchup
Marinara Sauce
Mayonnaise
Mustard
Peanut Butter
Ranch Dressing
Soy Sauce
Taco Seasoning
Tartar Sauce
Thai Marinade
Thousand Island Dressing
Tzatziki Sauce
Vegetable Broth
Worcestershire Sauce
Yogurt Dressing

Chapter 8: Snacks and Desserts

Apple Crumb Cake Muffins
Carrot Dip
Cauliflower Rice
Fiesta Dip
Macaroni & Cheese

Mozzarella Sticks
Peanut Butter Bars
Potato Salad
Red Pepper Hummus
Rice Pudding
South American Guacamole
Stuffed Mushrooms
Tomato Salsa
Trail Mix

Made in the
USA
Middletown, DE